KALEIDOSCOPE

Macrobiotic Articles, Essays, and Lectures 1979-1985

Herman Aihara

George Ohsawa Macrobiotic Foundation
Oroville, California

Mr. Aihara's works include:

Macrobiotics: An Invitation – June 1971
Milk – A Myth of Civilization – November 1971
Seven Macrobiotic Principles – January 1973
Soybean Diet – November 1974
Learning From Salmon – July 1980
Basic Macrobiotics – April 1985
Acid and Alkaline, Revised Edition – February 1986
Kaleidoscope – February 1986

Front cover photograph:
Spectral Light Painting © by Alex Nicoloff, Berkeley, California

Back cover photograph:
Mari Kennedy, Portland, Oregon

Illustrations:
Elizabeth Weil, El Cerrito, California

Library of Congress Catalog Card Number: 86-80031
ISBN 0-918860-37-7

Preface

For many of its early years in this country, macrobiotics was thought by some, especially in the mass media, to be a strange Asian dietary practice whose proponents graduated eventually to eating nothing but brown rice. During the sixties a few fanatics expanded this to include psychedelic or other drugs. Later, it was: "Macrobiotics? Oh, that's tofu, right?"

Today it's clear that the extensive techniques of macrobiotic cuisine preceded and have even influenced the current cuisine movement. Any experienced macrobiotic cook has long been ideally equipped in the preparation of many natural foods now rapidly gaining repute as health-giving and delectable.

But however essential the foods may be, the sublime concept of yin and yang, with its endless applications, remains the jewel of this teaching. And there is no one more qualified than Herman Aihara to explore the facets of this traditional wisdom – the wisdom that realizes nothing stays the same, everything alternates, not chaotically but with certain orderliness. Many people mention the principle of yin and yang, macrobiotic teachers included, but it would be hard to find anyone else living today who has delved as deeply into the subject.

In this regard he is the logical successor to George Ohsawa; he began studying under him in 1941 and continued as his translator, editor, and emissary until Ohsawa's passing in 1966, eventually founding the George Ohsawa Macrobiotic

Foundation in 1970. Today, he carries the Ohsawa spirit closely. If, in reading this book, you feel the student speaks of his teacher reverently (but with common sense) and frequently, you can understand why. In many ways he took up where Ohsawa left off. The student became the teacher but remained a student. He has also brought macrobiotics up to date, ignoring not even the smallest item of interest in current events. Ohsawa would have done the same.

A native of Japan living in the United States since 1952, Herman Aihara is an engineer, scientist, philosopher, and teacher who has written articles for the Foundation's monthly newsletters and for other publications with illumination on a diverse range of subjects for the past twenty-five years. He has always had something unique to say not only on health issues but also politics, business, the economy, human relationships, philosophy, and spirituality. Subscribers eagerly await his fresh and original thought with every issue, yet his readership has been relatively limited to this audience; evidently, today's popular press still thinks of macrobiotics as brown rice, whereas its real basis lies in what founder Ohsawa dubbed 'the unique principle' (yin and yang) – a physical interpretation of the ancient Chinese metaphysical system of natural balance. Herman goes a long way toward correcting this problem. "If you become attached to brown rice," he says, "you must give up brown rice too."

However, "give it up" does not mean forever, and this is one of the many examples of confusion when Eastern thought meets Western mind. Herman and Cornellia tell the story of a macrobiotic student who asked their advice on a dietary question of yin and yang. When they gave another lecture in that person's area some time later – a year or so – they found the person still following the same advice! "Just try for a while," they laughed, surprised at the static thinking. In the same way, they have been compelled to spell out such things as how much salt to use in cookbook recipes, having realized that this is the Western way. I hope Herman's sense of flexibility is conveyed in the pages of this book, for that is one of his greatest and most valuable lessons.

In 1980 we at the Foundation collected many prior Aihara writings in a volume called *Learning From Salmon*, named for one of its essay titles. During the ensuing six years, Herman has become even more prolific, clarifying his macrobiotic concepts in a matured and further defined writing style. The present volume represents a compilation of his newer articles, arranged this time in approximately chronological order instead of a composed pattern.

It has been, and is, a pleasure and an honor to work on these articles. It's a rare opportunity to learn from Herman while helping to clarify his meanings and expression. I thank him here for giving me this chance.

Like the earlier collection, this book is easy to read; essays can be chosen for their varying length and subject matter. The format is nondemanding of your time – there are only one or two longer pieces – but it invites steady unfoldment of the author's way of thinking. Most of the articles have appeared in Foundation newsletters (*GOMF News*, February 1979 to February 1984, and *Macrobiotics Today*, March 1984 to July 1985) and a few, noted by season rather than month, were published in *Macromuse*, the Washington, D.C. area quarterly.

"The Essence of Macrobiotics" I transcribed verbatim from one of Herman's animated lectures at his annual macrobiotic summer camp in the Sierras ("A Night at Vega," "How to Overcome Fear," "Thoughts on Marriage," and "Holding On and Letting Go" were also taken from lectures) and the "Nei Ching" translation is not exactly an article by him but we decided to include it anyway for its value. Some of the entries, such as the trip diaries, New Year's messages, and Ohsawa memorials, were intended as letters to Foundation members, but there was always that pearl of wisdom in each one that made it worth including here.

Herman writes all his articles in English with a strong command of the language; I've learned so much about writing from him. Still there are a few meanings that one may question. For example, the word 'happiness'. Why is it so often cited as a macrobiotic goal? Is this the simple happiness that Webster's defines as meaning "pleasurable satisfaction" or suggesting "a dazed irresponsible state . . . enthusiastic to the point of obsession"? Could this be the ultimate aim of macrobiotics, as some topics or wordings seem to suggest?

Hardly. But, seeing constant repetition of the term, one might be inclined to think so unless a deeper meaning be uncovered.

Explaining further the Ohsawa and Aihara usage of 'happy', Webster's also offers: "A state of well-being and contentment . . . notably well-adapted or fitting." A deeper overall satisfaction comes to mind ("Happy even when sick," Herman says), indicating a larger sense of joy in life that can of course include the usual kind of happiness. And what better key to this happiness than the little compass of yin and yang which teaches the art of adaptability? Herman's friend, the "rare, happy cancer patient," was 'happy' because she would have been willing to repeat her life exactly the same, without any changes.

Ohsawa's method of showing the inclusiveness of his all-embracing or 'eternal happiness' lies within the structure of the seven levels of judgment. His notion of 'supreme judgment', to which one can 'tune in' via the cosmic channel of higher functioning, is an all-inclusive state to be cherished and encouraged despite our tendency to dwell in the lower, non-absolute, relative worlds of judgment.

In the closing article here, "Supreme Judgment," Herman makes an important point when he explains that even brief experiences of 'supreme judgment' are powerful and healing. Much in the same way that he illuminates the yin and yang idea as an in-flux situation (that is, not seeing life a pendulum but rather things changing, changing back, and then changing some more), he eliminates the danger of thinking that one obtains supreme judgment and stays there, or one does not.

And the macrobiotic usage of 'judgment' itself calls for examination under the macro microscope too; we are not talking about judgmental opinions, but about consciousness, awareness, and evalution by the fine capacities of discernment. Ohsawa referred to the 'veiled judgment' of modern humanity, a term which nearly self-explains his meaning for the verb 'to judge.'

But how to obtain this supreme judgment?

Become trustworthy and respected; maintain good balance in health; be humble in all activities; and, most important, remain as all-embracing, as inclusive as possible. Who can qualify for these conditions? The closest candidate is Herman Aihara, the one who was impressed forty years ago by the wisdom and energy of his teacher and inspiration, George Ohsawa, and who so faithfully but unfanatically carries on these ideals for his own students in the Western world and around the globe.

Sandy Rothman
November 1985

From the Author

A title for this book was discussed one day this autumn at the Foundation office. *Macrobiotic Journal* was one title advised. It is a good name but I wasn't satisfied because it sounds too normal, no excitement. I was thinking a few days. And then I got the name – *Macrobiotic Kaleidoscope*. I announced it at the staff meeting. They liked the name very much. However, I realized it was too long, so I agreed to change it to just *Kaleidoscope*. In Greek, *kalos* is "beautiful" and *eidos* means "form". Therefore, a kaleidoscope is an instrument that shows beautiful forms.

When I was a college student I read a book called *Kaleidoscope* written by a famous scientist named T. Terada. He was also famous as a writer and haiku poet but not so much as a provoker of Japanese language. He supported an idea that Japanese should be written in the Roman alphabet so that it could be typed by typewriter easily. George Ohsawa had the same idea. I am not sure whether Ohsawa learned the idea from Dr. Terada or not. In any event, Ohsawa admired him. When I was living in New York City, Ohsawa visited the United States and stayed at my apartment. On one occasion, I mentioned my admiration for Terada's writing. As soon as Ohsawa returned to Tokyo, he sent me a whole set of Dr. Terada's works, which I treasure among my most precious books.

His *Kaleidoscope* includes many short articles, observations on natural phenomena, social matters, and human behavior, and scientific reports. What made me interested in his writing was his objective view and lack of emotion in his opinion. His style is the result of his haiku training. Haiku is a seventeen-syllable poem which is the shortest form of poetry. However, the uniqueness of haiku is not its short form but its rule of expression.

The rule of haiku is: it must express location, season, and nature. In other words, haiku must express space, time, and the orderliness of nature in seventeen syllables. Terada was a master of haiku; therefore, his writing was objective and yet hitting the point.

My *Kaleidoscope* is the accumulation of my writings from *GOMF News, Macrobiotics Today,* and *Macromuse* over the past six years, expressing my macrobiotic opinion on various subjects such as social issues, political and economic matters, and health. When I wrote, I tried to be as good as Dr. Terada. I am not sure I could achieve that aim or not. However, after I read all these articles, I felt I was looking in a kaleidoscope. In fact, macrobiotics is an instrument to judge and think on natural and social phenomena with yin and yang as the two mirrors. These two mirrors show ever-changing beautiful forms. It is my greatest pleasure if I ever could give you kaleidoscopic images, made of the two mirrors of yin and yang, by this book, so that your view of life is more colorful and meaningful.

I would like to thank the many who helped in producing this book. For the original editing of the articles: Sandy Rothman, Kevin Meutsch, Gerry Thompson, and Stan Hodson. The final editing was done by Sandy Rothman with help from Carl Ferre, who was also responsible for text design and production. I wish also to thank Sandy for the cover concept, Sylvia Zuck for typesetting, Julia Ferre for proofreading, and Stan Hodson for work on the index.

Contents

New Year's Message, 1980

Over the Western Sea hither
from Nippon come,
Courteous, the swart-cheek'd
two sworded envoys
Leaning back in their open
barouches, bare headed
impassive,
Ride to-day through Manhattan.

Thus Walt Whitman saluted seventy-seven Japanese samurai on June 17, 1860, when the biggest crowds of New Yorkers ever on Broadway welcomed the visitors, 120 years ago.

Vice Ambassador Awaji No-Kami Muragaki said in his diary:

> It was 2:00 p.m. when our boat arrived in New York harbor, where many ships were anchored and thousands of spectators were waiting at the piers. We paraded on a big street following American battalions. It was said that 8000 soldiers and officers of 12 battalions attended the parade. Thousands of civilians attended. Both sides of the road were filled with people welcoming us – there was no room left at all. We arrived at the hotel in late evening. It was a six story building and very luxurious. Every window was decorated with Japanese flags. Children also welcomed us with Japanese flags on hand. . .

1

According to the record, every window and every roof was full of people who wanted to see the strange Japanese they had never heard of, much less seen, before. Shrewd store owners were charging $1.00 per seat which they quickly built in front of their shops for this parade.

The New York Times reported that the city of New York spent $91,380 for the fourteen-day reception for the seventy-seven samurai. If evaluated by today's standards, it would be close to a million dollars.

The Japanese Embassy came to America to exchange documents pertaining to the Treaty of Amity and Commerce between the governments of the United States and Japan, represented by the head of the Embassy, Masaaki Shinmi.

Since the welcoming enthusiasm displayed by the Americans for the Japanese Embassy was merely a burst of curiosity, the event did not much increase American interest in Japan. However, the Japanese, who had not been contacted for three hundred years at that time, acquired a tremendous interest in America and Americans. Japanese students, scholars, politicians, and merchants started to visit here. About a hundred years ago, on May 27, 1869, the first group of immigrants arrived in the United States. They settled in Gold Hill, California, and set up the Wakamatsu Tea and Silk Farm Colony. Since then, Japanese immigrants and visitors have increased every year. At the end of 1970 the Japanese population in the States was 591,290. They are the second largest race, excluding the white and black races, next to the Indian. (*The Japanese in America 1843-1973*, compiled by Masako Herman, Oceana Publications, 1974.)

After the two countries exchanged treaties, the Japanese learned Western science, technology, and culture from the Americans with much enthusiasm. However, the two nations didn't know each other well until World War II when Japan learned enough about Western weaponry and thought her industry was big enough to fight against the United States and European countries.

Following World War II, the relationship between the two nations was most interesting. Losing many young male workers at the front and at home, Japan suffered from lack of housing, clothing, and foods – except expensive black market goods – and had no schools, no transportation system, and no amusements. This hardship, especially the shortage of food, was the main cause for Japan's development as the world's number one industrial country. Young Japanese became the most materialistic, economic-minded people. Contrary to Japan, industry in the United States increased due to the war, which demanded many weapons, and there was much profit. America was rich and life was comfortable. This richness and comfort produced a lazy, intellectual, and metaphysical youth. Americans became more and more interested in learning Oriental philosophy, culture, medicine, and way of life.

Just as this trend started, exactly one hundred years after the first samurai visited here, a neatly-dressed and deeply-voiced Japanese gentleman was welcomed by about a hundred well-educated, middle-class Americans at the New Horizon Summer Camp in Long Island, New York. His name was George Ohsawa, westernized from his Japanese name Yukikazu Sakurazawa. He gave lectures and consultations several hours every day for two months. He had tremendous knowledge, intelligence, and humor. His speech was very witty, amusing, and heart penetrating. He conducted meetings with question after question. The more intellectual the listeners, the more ignorant they realized themselves to be. Whoever listened to him was convinced of his diet and philosophy; soon he was always surrounded by as many fanatic, enthusiastic students in America as he had been in Europe.

The reason Americans listened to George Ohsawa and became interested in macrobiotics was not merely from curiosity: they did so on matters of life and death. When we have enough money, food, clothes, homes, and conveniences for living, we start looking for something else – the moon, space, the environment, pollution, etc. – and we find enough time to investigate what we have done in the so-called twentieth century civilization. Contrary to the belief that medical clinics and hospitals were so developed that man would soon be free from sickness, we discover in reality that modern medicine has no solution to cancer, heart disease, and other degenerative illnesses. Ohsawa explained the cause of these modern diseases and told how to attain health, curing incurable diseases with the simplest diet.

It was an atomic bomb for Americans. It was too powerful a knowledge, too much change of lifestyle for most Americans. Some, misguided by an ignorant and unjust news media, left the macrobiotic diet when a few unfortunate events happened. However, justice cannot be stopped and the true value of macrobiotics cannot be hidden. It will be more and more practiced in the States. The practice of macrobiotics, it seems to me, is a meeting of East and West. In other words, we are becoming Man instead of Japanese, Chinese, American, white or black.

So far, East and West have met at the sensorial, sentimental, and intellectual levels. The rest of the twentieth century will be a trial for the East and the West: they must meet at higher levels of judgment such as the religious, social, economic, and ultimate concepts of life.

In the world situation today the East cannot escape the influence of the West. The West cannot live even a day without the influence of the East. The world literally is one. This is due to science, technology, industry, communication, and transportation. However, the sciences of biology, physiology, and medicine are so undeveloped that there are many questions in life. We don't know our origin; why we are as we are; where we are going; how our body works, etc. Therefore we don't really know our neighbors or other people. The problems are bigger and deeper when it comes to our consciousness or mind. Towards the understanding of consciousness or mind we have nothing but confusion, mystery, and questions. We don't know how we think, how brain cells are made for thinking or if that is where thinking is done. We don't know how we remember; how emotions such as anger, joy, or resentment are made; where and how we create our concept of life; what is happiness, justice, etc.

Since we don't know our mind, how it works and what it is made of, it is difficult to understand and communicate with others. Making problems more difficult, there are language barriers: every nationality speaks a different language. The real understanding of any new language, if not impossible, may take more than twenty years of hard study.

Furthermore, we have prejudices and different backgrounds in education, culture, customs and family traditions – and we have exclusivity. These things make us egoistic and create separation between people. This exclusivity and what Ohsawa called arrogance seem to me the fundamental problems of humanity.

The concept of yin and yang will be a great help in the further development of biology, physiology, and medicine because nature is made by the two forces of yin and yang, and our body is a part of nature. Therefore, in the coming years I will continue to study, write, and lecture on these subjects and the Foundation will publish books which will promote this understanding.

For our consciousness, mind, exclusivity, and arrogance Ohsawa gave us an excellent education. However, I am not as good as Ohsawa. I am just praying I can be a man of nonexclusivity and no arrogance. After a few years, Cornellia and I will start Vega Institute again where I hope we can more intensively improve our consciousness and spirituality together.

I hope the year of 1980 is a great and happy one for all of you.

Lecture Trip in Europe

London

The first European Macrobiotic Congress was held during November 1978, at the Community Health Foundation in London. With its restaurant, food shop, and many lecture halls, this building served well for the meeting. Originally the Congress had been scheduled for Ghent and the sudden change was difficult. However, the Congress was well organized.

About two hundred macrobiotic leaders from Europe and some from the United States gathered to honor Mrs. Lima Ohsawa and Shuzo Okada. The meeting started with a meditation in memory of George Ohsawa whose picture was displayed on the wall. Michio Kushi gave the opening speech saying that a North American Macrobiotic Congress will be held in 1979, and will be followed by a Congress in South America, and then one in Asia.

The next day, I was asked to give a speech after Lima Ohsawa's and Shuzo Okada's speeches. I said:

"Michio Kushi will organize similar congresses in North America, South America, and Asia. This is a great idea. Many will be stimulated and observe a macrobiotic diet. However, I see two difficulties in this movement. One is a jealous mentality among leaders. A less popular leader will be jealous of another who is more popular. This jealousy will create resentments and be a hazard to a peaceful mind. Even though one peaceful world is realized, if each one is not peaceful, how good is such a world.

"Another problem concerns food distribution. The macrobiotic movement is related to food – the special kinds of food which cannot be bought at a regular market. Therefore, food distribution is one of the activities of macrobiotics as well as a source of income for some. Many macrobiotic followers as well as some others conduct the macrobiotic food businesses. Doing business can create a greedy mentality and an exclusive ego, which is not the character macrobiotics aims to achieve. If this happens, resentment, gossip, tricks, even arrogance will be observed among macrobiotic people. We have to be humble and reflect more in order to succeed in such a movement."

Amsterdam

On November 14th in the evening, I left London for Amsterdam with Ineke Niermeyer, who had been at Vega two years ago with her husband and two children. Early the next morning, we arrived at the Holland port. The weather was nice, but chilly. We arrived at Amsterdam after a two-hour ride on the train. The town was busy and active, and very clean.

The East West Center, which was organized eight years ago by Adelbert Nelissen, is a big house facing a canal. It consists of a big lecture hall, an exercise hall, a food store, a printing room, a camera room, a dining room, several dormitories and Adelbert's family room. They own eight stores, bakeries and the center house. They bake one ton of bread every day using flour ground by windmill. It seems to me to be one of the best organized centers in Europe.

I started the first night's lecture at 8:00 p.m. with about seventy people attending. They were mostly between twenty and thirty years of age. I talked about how I met Ohsawa, and about my difficulty with the Immigration Law. I finished around 10:30 p.m.

On November 16th, Abe Nakamura took me to his home in Dusseldorf – a two-hour drive. His business has been well established in Germany. However, he is losing his customers to Michio's students who are opening several stores in the same town. Such things make him reluctant to help Michio. I see such mentality among the Japanese macrobiotic leaders in Europe. This problem relates to their living income, so it is difficult to solve.

That night, I spoke about the macrobiotic diet, physiology, yin yang principles, balancing sodium and potassium, and balancing acid and alkaline.

On the 17th, I talked about balancing hormones, nervous systems, and Selye's stress theory, concluding that we will not have absolute peace of mind unless we reach complete gratitude and absolute faith in the order of the universe.

On the 18th, the meeting started in the morning. I talked about the spiralic concept of man. Real man is the whole universe. Macrobiotic means becoming such a person. During the afternoon, I taught Sotai exercise, which they enjoyed very much. Then I gave palm diagnosis of family and marriage, and palm reading. This created a strong curiosity – everyone came around me asking me to read their palms.

Antwerp

Outside the station, Mr. Rik Vermuyten, whom I had met in London, was waiting for me. He drove me to the macrobiotic restaurant in Antwerp, where Mr. and Mrs. Peter Doggen and two other couples and I had a Sunday lunch.

After lunch, I was guided to Peter's home, which houses a macrobiotic bakery. The store and the center are situated in different locations. The center is much smaller than Amsterdam's center but contains a restaurant, office, lecture hall, and dormitories.

The meeting started at 8:00 p.m. Since there are many family troubles there, I was asked to talk about how to unite the family. About fifty people came; most were family people and were older than those attending in Amsterdam. They responded well. The leaders of macrobiotics in Antwerp are mostly family people in their thirties.

London

The next morning, Peter took me to a nearby airport, and from there I flew back to London. I went to the Community Health Foundation in the evening by subway. Bill Tara greeted me and we dined together.

The audiences were much younger in London – most of them in their early twenties. I talked on similar subjects which I had talked about in Amsterdam. By the third day, many asked questions and there was much discussion.

Bologna

On November 24th, I arrived in Bologna and was welcomed by a well-dressed Italian youth, Alois Grassani. The center, a three-story building, had a food shop which was very crowded, kitchen, dining rooms, and offices. They serve lunch and dinner self-service style. There, I met an American girl from Philadelphia, and she guided me to their publishing and business offices in a separate building. They publish a bi-monthly magazine, *Ting*, in three languages – Italian, French, and English. These are well edited, documented, and printed on expensive paper. The distribution and retailing of macrobiotic foods supports these publications.

They don't call their activity 'macrobiotics', but rather, '*A New Way*'. Also, they have a different idea for cooking. Instead of cooking foods on fire the conventional way, they cook grains, beans, and vegetables on fire for only fifteen minutes and then cover with a blanket for one to two hours.

I tasted foods prepared this way. The beans were excellent. Grains were not bad, but could be better. They said that vegetables are better cooked the conventional way. This method of cooking may be good in California, Nevada, Arizona, or Texas, where the temperatures are high. They do this to save energy and for the psychological reason that fire creates ego emotion. I advised them that this system may be good for yang people, but may be not so good for yin people who need more yang (fire) preparation.

My lecture was supposed to start at 10:00 a.m., but did not actually start until 10:30. They said that this is Italian time. I said, "this is Japanese time, too," and they laughed. At noon, we had a break and started again at 2:00. The lecture ended at 6:00 and at 8:00 we started again. It was 10:00 p.m. before I finished the long day.

On the 26th, the meeting started at 12 noon and lasted until 6:00 p.m. At the end of the lecture, I gave palm diagnosis and fortunetelling – many came around me after the lecture. That night, I was invited to a party which was organized by workers of the center. About twenty people and some friends from other centers gathered. When they began to gossip about macrobiotic centers in Europe, the leader of this center, Alois, asked them to stop such talking. He seems to have understood my message during the two days of lectures.

On November 27th, I gave consultations all morning. That afternoon, Mauro and Alois took me to their new house outside Bologna, overlooking the green hills of northern Italy. They, the center members, are renting a seven-bedroom remodeled house very cheaply. Several families will move in soon. They even plan to have a summer camp there this coming year.

Since I had left my raincoat on the train near Paris, the center people bought one for me and gave it as a present. Later, it helped me very much in the cold temperatures of France, Belgium, and England.

Paris

The train arrived at the Lyon Station in Paris on time. I took a taxi to the Tenryu Institute where I was greeted by Clim Yoshimi and Francoise Riviere. Tenryu rents three buildings and operates a store, lecture room, office, and restaurant. They are a well-established business. As everywhere else, their food business supports the publishing of a magazine. The monthly publication here is called *Principe Unique* (Unique Principle), one of the names Ohsawa coined to explain his philosophy.

About twenty people gathered for my lecture that night. Most of them were senior macrobiotic students in France. I talked about macrobiotic history in the United States, especially on the West Coast. Afterwards we enjoyed a midnight dinner at a Paris seafood restaurant, proving that macrobiotic people are great eaters.

The next day, Clim took me to Mr. Loc's bookstore, which is small but has a big offset press and process camera on the second floor. After leaving the bookstore, I visited the *Journal Le Compas*. Mr. Philippe Pred'Homme, editor of the journal, said that the *Compas* circulates only 6000 copies quarterly. Therefore, the paper not only doesn't make money, but also doesn't pay wages at all. Three Frenchmen and one woman work free. I appreciate their devoted attitude toward macrobiotics. Many such contributors have made macrobiotics what it is today.

Clim and I had dinner at a Japanese restaurant with two other oldtime macrobiotic friends from Japan and found that

Japanese foods are very popular in Paris. Then we went to a famous cafe, Dome, to talk more. We joked, laughed, and talked until closing time, 2:00 a.m., with only two cups of coffee each. The cost was $10, so Paris is quite expensive.

Ghent

The next morning, the last day of November, Clim drove me to Ghent. He took me to the Lima factory, where I had worked for a while seventeen years ago after I had been deported by the U.S. government. Today the Lima factory is so big and well established. They bake five tons of bread every day by wood fire. All production, such as the packaging of grain, flour, miso, and tamari, is done by automation. To my surprise, they have a laboratory where they can inspect foods for insecticides, coloring, chemicals, etc. They can even distinguish kuzu from arrowroot.

After visiting the Lima factory, Clim took me to his new center which he rented recently. It is located in front of the Ghent train station and has four stories. He is planning to leave Tenryu and work in this center solely to make a food store, give cooking classes and lectures, and to rent rooms. He will be very active and much happier in the coming years. I hope he will become a big leader of macrobiotics in Europe as well as the world.

Conclusion

On December 1st, Abe Nakamura visited me again at the Brussels Airport. We talked about many subjects, including such questions as: How consciousness creates or stimulates hormone production, especially acetylcholine? Why grains are the main food of man? The change of gravitation on the earth? This is the foundation of my view that there was a stone civilization on earth about six thousand or more years ago.

We had a hard time saying goodbye after seeing each other for the first time in seventeen years. Time had passed quickly – my three-week trip to Europe was over. I made a lot of friends and was invited back by many centers.

European macrobiotics exceeds macrobiotics in America in quantity; however, I do not know about quality. Macrobiotic students are more concentrated than those in America. They stimulate each other more and thus develop faster than in America. European macrobiotic students are in two classes, senior and beginner; in America they seem to fit in between. Thus, European macrobiotics and American macrobiotics will mix well, and will create a better macrobiotic movement. For this, we need to develop better lines of communication.

Jonestown

Almost ending 1978, the world was shocked at hearing of a mass murder/suicide by members of the People's Temple in Guyana. Humanity has not experienced such a thing in recent history. Nine hundred and twelve people followed the order of a madman in whom they believed as God, and committed suicide. I couldn't understand why almost a thousand people killed themselves like computer-programmed robots. They lost their own judgment and will to live.

However, there is no accident in this world. Everything has a cause. What caused this mass murder/suicide? Of the 912, the majority were black people. Black people have been slaves, unfree, poor, and unhappy. Therefore they have been looking for anything that will help them. Because of this, they believed in Jim Jones as a prophet. Jones seemed to them a savior who preached and promised a land where everyone would be equal in life as they were in the eyes of the Lord.

Jim Jones was such a good speaker that his followers trusted him more and more. As their trust in him increased, they called him 'Father', asking him to heal their ills. Jones obliged by giving them palm healing which may have come from his instinctive judgment. Soon they called him 'prophet'. The more faithful they became, the more power Jones had. Finally, Jones claimed himself as the messiah of black people.

When the People's Temple membership reached about

five hundred he moved to northern California, to the Mendocino County Seat, Ukiah. This move may have begun the deadly march towards the mass murder/suicide. If he had not moved, it may never have happened. I strongly believe so because after he moved to California, he started to take drugs – 'speed'. Why did he start to take speed? Because he had so much to do. "Some hundred persons eventually made the journey. Houses had to be rented for them. Jobs had to be found for those who could work," said Phil Tracy in the December 18th (1978) issue of *New West* magazine.

This reminded me of 1961 when sixteen macrobiotic families moved from New York City to Chico, California. After moving to Chico they started Chico-San, Inc., and began the Ohsawa Foundation of Chico. They were the first macrobiotic community and macrobiotic foods manufacturer in this country. This group was very faithful to its leader, George Ohsawa, as were the members of the People's Temple to their leader, Jim Jones. However, one big difference between them is that the macrobiotic group didn't take any drugs.

Reporting on this, *New West* said:

> Shortly after reaching northern California Jones began taking amphetamines to help himself keep up the pace. A man with a congregation convinced he was God addicted himself to one of the deadliest mind-distorting drugs available. Later, it was rumored, friendly doctors in the Mendocino area provided the drugs by prescription. . . . Jones began to visit the San Francisco Bay Area, attending various civic and protest rallies, gradually picking up on the latest New Left theories. Jones came to believe that his mission was to emulate not Christ, but Lenin or Mao Tse-tung. He was going to create a brand new social order based on racial equality, revolutionary communalism and sexual liberation.

From this time on, probably around 1970, Jones's madness became more and more apparent and his erratic actions and paranoid behavior increased, according to *New West:*

> Members were informed that their marriages and sex-
> ual partnerships were corrupt. Husbands and wives
> were forced to sleep with different partners. Spying was
> systematized. Jones announced that government agents
> were trying to penetrate the planning commission, and
> that thereafter each member should be prepared to
> inform him as to the actions and statements of any other
> member. . . . Shortly after Martin Luther King was
> killed, Jones faked his own assassination with the help
> of an aide who fired blank cartridges and a Baggie full of
> chicken blood to stain his shirt. Jones reappeared an
> hour later, claiming he had raised himself from the
> dead. After that, planning commission members
> dressed in costume and makeup would collapse 'dead'
> at a prearranged signal, and be 'brought back to life' by
> Jones. These antics eventually attracted the attention of
> the *San Francisco Examiner*'s then religious editor; in
> September of 1972 he wrote a series of articles on
> Jones's healing powers. But Jones was able to squelch
> any follow-up investigation by organizing a massive
> letter-writing and picket-line campaign against the
> paper.

Even though Jones's behavior became so abnormal, many of
the blacks still believed Jones was God – even when he started
telling them there was no God and that he was the reincarnation of Lenin. As Jones increased his self-made psychological
fear and distortion of social order in the U.S., he demanded
that members prepare to move to a new Promised Land, the
Marxist republic of Guyana, South America, in order to
escape the "fascist dictatorship" of America's government.

After collecting an enormous amount of materials and
money, they moved to Guyana . . . and finally, Jones became
insane and asked members to follow him toward the end of life.

I understand that the insanity of Jones was caused by the use
of drugs. But it is hard to understand why the black people

believed in Jones so faithfully. They died for what? What shall we learn from their action? Probably nobody can explain except the ones who died. The karma from ancestors and from their own deeds of the past helped to cause this fatal action. High consumption of sugar creates a strongly submissive, passive, and innocent character. In my speculation, Jones's use of drugs and the black members' high consumption of sugar would be the immediate major causes leading to this tragedy.

Changing China

"China is already a great power, and whether the next three decades will be a cold or a hot war, nothing can stop her now. By the year 2001 she will be a powerful industrial socialist state," said Suyin Han in her book *China in the Year 2001* (Basic Books, 1967). Her prediction may be right but she may not be expecting the way China will industrialize. Nobody in the world may have expected such a sudden change in the Chinese attitude, opening the gate to the exchange of culture, science, technology, and economy.

"The project is vast, daring and unique in history. How could there be a precedent for turning one billion people so sharply in their course, for leading one-quarter of mankind out of dogmatic isolation into the late 20th century and the life of the rest of the planet?" (*Time* magazine, January 1, 1979). This is one of the biggest decisions made by humans in this century. This decision will change world history like Hitler and Tojo did in starting World War II.

"It is difficult for Westerners to understand how so vast a population can psychologically reverse itself so quickly. But the Chinese character instinctively believes that life constantly swings between extremes. They said that the momentum of history was ever thus: the empire, long divided, must unite; long united, must divide. In any case, the Chinese leaders are preparing for a reversal of nearly everything that Mao Tse-tung taught. . ." A few years ago, if a farmer was asked about the most important factor in increasing rice production, he would answer automatically: "Mastering the thought of Chairman Mao." Now he is more likely to respond: "More chemical fertilizer" (*Time*).

Almost thirty years after the People's Republic was founded in 1949, Chinese leaders realized that some of Mao's thought on how to develop China was wrong. The main mistake was his Cultural Revolution, which shut China off from the rest of the world. It caused Chinese agriculture to remain primitive so that farmers could not produce enough grain for their people, and kept the Chinese military machinery so primitive that it is at least twenty years behind that of the superpowers. It eliminated intellectuals, so the development of science and technology was stopped for twenty years.

In order to correct these mistakes, Chinese Vice Premier Teng Hsiao-p'ing was brave and strong enough to begin changing Mao's policy, which has been like a Bible in the way of life for one billion Chinese. Teng called this movement the Four Modernizations – an attempt to simultaneously improve agriculture, industry, science/technology, and defense. The project is so unusual, and historically unique, that we may compare it only to the Japanese and German development after World War II or to the American industrialization following World War I.

Having one of the oldest histories of civilization and culture and the biggest population on this planet, and having closed its gates to other countries for such a long time, China has been considered a sleeping tiger. Even Napoleon was afraid to wake her. Now this sleeping tiger has awakened.

Due to its vast resources and population, China has great potential for a future in economy, technology, and industry. In 1978 China decided to learn all modern technology, develop its own industry, and fully cultivate its own natural resources.

This will bring a tremendous influence to the world, including the merchandise market, airline routes, news media, TV shows, science, politics, and especially the military balance sheets of the world.

According to *U.S. News & World Report* (December 11, 1978), the true goal of the Four Modernizations can be summarized: To oppose or frustrate the Soviet Union everywhere and at all levels. This view was confirmed in an interview with Teng Hsiao-p'ing by *Time* editor-in-chief Hedley Donovan. Teng answered Donovan's question on Soviet policies, saying:

> The nuclear arsenal of the Soviet Union and the constant development of their strategic weapons means that we can say the Soviet Union is already on a par with the U.S. The Soviet military budget takes up around 20% of the gross national product. What does one do with all these things? With no war going on, it has increased its standing army in three years from 3 million to 4 million men. What does one do that for? If one has so many things in one's hands, the day will come when one's fingers begin to itch. You can't eat those materials or wear them. You must use them somehow. We've already been through two world wars, and both started from small incidents . . . We consider that the true hotbed of war is the Soviet Union, not the U.S.

Chinese leaders are urging the promotion of the New Long March to protect against aggressive Russian militarism. However, in my opinion, Teng and the Chinese leaders are not so afraid of the Russians, but are using antagonism against Russia as their reason to change Mao's policy, so long and faithfully followed by a billion Chinese. Teng and other leaders know now that if they don't change Mao's policy, Chinese communism will completely fail in supporting their people. So, Chinese leaders are changing Mao's policy. However, many people may find it difficult to understand the reason. Therefore, Teng is telling the people that China has to modernize her industry, agriculture, technology, and defense systems in order to protect against Russian militarism, even though they have to ask the help of capitalist countries.

China's new policy to open up its gate and share with other countries toward world peace and prosperity is a wonderful idea. I admire Teng's judgment and courage. However, some of his ideas cause me to worry. He is making the same big mistake made by leaders of other industrialized countries if he introduces chemical fertilizers and insecticides in Chinese farming.

He must study recent developments in organic gardening and the atomic transmutation theory so that the green earth of China will not be spoiled by giving it chemical fertilizer.

Another important suggestion, to me, for his New Long March is: Don't use sugar in people's diet. *Time* reported that the Chinese government gave Coca-Cola exclusive rights to sell in the People's Republic. What sad news. If this is true, the People's Republic of China is walking the same road towards self-destruction as many other countries, under the name of high civilization or industrialization. The Chinese leaders must be aware that all 'civilized' countries have higher rates of high and low blood pressure, multiple sclerosis, cancer, and diabetes – that is to say, all the so-called degenerative diseases. The cause of these diseases, according to Oriental medicine, is the excessive use of refined and processed foods, high fat foods, extremely yin foods such as sugar, and chemical additives such as saccharin, dyes, and preservatives.

Most scientists disagree with this view nowadays – perhaps because they are working for food manufacturing companies. However, a few honest and sincere scientists are expressing the idea that there is a link between degenerative diseases and the use of sugar and chemicals mentioned above. There are thousands of books and other literature concerning this subject published in many languages if not Chinese. I sincerely hope

the Chinese leaders investigate and study the destructive function of chemicals and sugar before they introduce them into
their farming and food importing and manufacturing.

I divinated the present situation of the New Long March of
China with the *I-Ching*. The hexagram (which includes part of
Teng's name) appeared as (9) 小畜 ☰☴ Hsaio Ch'u: The tam-
ing power of the small. "In the Image it is the wind blowing
across the sky. The wind restrains the clouds . . . and makes
them grow dense, but as yet is not strong enough to turn them
to rain." (*The I-Ching*, Wilhelm/Barnes edition, Princeton
University Press, 1977.) There are some difficulties and problems in the present situation. The difficulties or clouds over-
casting China suggested by the hexagram are, in my opinion,
the policies of food and agriculture. (The rest is fine, as
expressed in the hexagram. Proceed with your policy with
confidence; you have only to correct policies on foods and
farming, exercising care in food manufacturing and farming
techniques.) If China observes its ancient wisdom to keep soil
free from chemicals and avoids too much refining and the use
of sugar or chemicals, the Chinese will maintain their health
and eventually succeed with their Four Modernizations. Otherwise, China will not only fail their Modernizations but also will
be attacked by Russia, which, being a northern country, is
more yang than China. According to the *I-Ching*:

> This image refers to the state of affairs in China at the
> time when King Wen, who came originally from the
> West, was in the East at the court of the reigning tyrant
> Chou Hsin. The moment for action on a large scale had
> not yet arrived. King Wen could not keep the tyrant in
> check by friendly persuasion. Hence the image of many
> clouds, promising moisture and blessing to the land,
> although as yet no rain falls. The situation is not favor-
> able; there is a prospect of ultimate success, but there
> are still obstacles in the way, and we can merely take
> preparatory measures.

Russia is the tyrant. China's New Long March will succeed only through the small means of friendly persuasion. The same book translates, "To carry out our purpose we need firm determination within and gentleness and adaptability in external relations." I see strong determination in Teng and gentleness in his attitude. China will succeed with the New Long March in most cases. However, I see a small failure which could destroy China in the future: that is to say, the introduction of chemicals and sugar in agriculture and foods.

April 1979

The Nei Ching, Chapter 1
A modern translation from the Japanese

There was a wise emperor who lived in China in ancient times called the Yellow Emperor. He was very smart. Even when he was a baby he already understood conversation. When he was a youth he was wise. When he was an adult, he had integrity and became a king. After his death, it is said, he rose to Heaven riding a dragon.

One day this Yellow Emperor asked his teacher Chi'Po, "I have heard that ancient people easily lived over a hundred years with vigor. However, modern people hardly live over fifty years. What makes this difference? Is this caused by climatic change or change in the way of life?"

Chi'Po answered, "Ancient wise men often taught people how to preserve life by advising to consult divination and astrology. In ancient times people lived according to the order of the universe. They controlled eating, had orderliness in living, and avoided extra stress and strain. Their body and mind were well balanced. Therefore they could live over a hundred years. Modern people, contrary to this, have no orderliness. They drink liquor and eat meat in excessive amounts, and make love in excess. They pursue the satisfaction of their desires and show no control in living. Therefore, they grow old in fifty years. If one avoids extra ego desires, one's spirit circulates through the whole body and the internal organs function well. Therefore we maintain blood circulation and kidney circulation (this includes maintenance of the sex organs and sex energy). Such persons can protect themselves from outside causes of sickness such as bacterial diseases.

"It is advisable to avoid too many commitments; doing a job just well enough to manage allows the mind to maintain peace and have less stress. Avoid extreme hard work so that metabolic energy and protective energy circulate well through the body. In other words, a man who has less ego desire lives with satisfaction. For such persons, pure and simple foods taste good, simple clothes are enough to wear, and one does not need or attract any high status. With such people, the poor don't envy the rich. The rich don't show off to the poor. As a result, the society will be well-mannered and peaceful. In such a society people live a happy life because they are not misled by false, temporary pleasures. Neither the fool, the wise, nor the smart have worry. This means they must have lived an orderly life without violating natural order. Therefore they could have lived over a hundred years."

The Yellow Emperor asked, "Why can we not bear children after a certain age? Is this just because of old age, or that we have used up our seed for children?"

Chi'Po replied, "At first I will speak about women: At the age of 7, a girl gains the energy of the kidneys. As a result, she has permanent teeth and abundant hair. At the age of 14, she begins the ability of sex, completes the front center meridian, develops the Blood Ocean of the eighth meridian, and has regular menstruation. Thus, the ability to bear children is completed. At the age of 21, the energy of the kidneys circulates evenly through the whole body and the last teeth grow. At the age of 28, having muscles and hair well developed, she reaches womanhood. At the age of 35, the clear yang meridian starts to deteriorate, causing wrinkles and falling of hair. At the age of 42, the large yang, the clear yang, and the small yang meridians deteriorate, causing lack of nutrition in the face;

therefore, wrinkles and grey hairs increase. At the age of 49, the front central meridian becomes hollow (empty inside) and the eighth meridian deteriorates, causing less blood. Therefore, menstruation and the ability to bear children stops. Then, function of the sexual organs deteriorates and finally she completely loses the ability to bear children.

"For men, the biorhythm changes by eight-year cycles. At the age of 8, the energy of the kidneys develops well, hair grows abundantly and the permanent teeth appear. At the age of 16, sex energy matures and he is fully manly. Therefore he is able to perform sex and create children. At the age of 24, the kidney energy (sex energy) circulates through the whole body, muscles grow well, and the last teeth appear, completing tooth growth. At the age of 32, having strong muscles, he is at the highest condition of manhood. At the age of 40, the sex energy starts to diminish, hair lessens, and the teeth deteriorate. At the age of 48, the circulation of yang energy becomes weaker, causing lack of nutrition in the face; this brings wrinkles to the face and grey hairs to the head. At the age of 56, the liver energy becomes weak and the muscles lose their ability of expansion and contraction. Kidney functions also deteriorate and he loses sex ability. The whole body undergoes so-called 'aging'. At the age of 64, teeth and hair fall out and do not grow again. Since teeth and hair are related to the kidneys, this means the kidneys are weak. The kidney is an organ which stores energy (*seiki*) which activates internal organs. The weak kidney means all internal organs are weak. In other words, he loses sex appetite, hair becomes grey, muscles become loose, feet are weak, and the body is rigid. Therefore, he is not able to produce children."

The Yellow Emperor asked, "However, sometimes old men have children. What is the cause of this?"

Chi'Po answered, "This is because he was born with especially strong kidneys so that energy circulated very well through the meridians. However, it will be a rare case that one has good sexual appetite after the age of forty-nine for women and sixty-four for men."

The Yellow Emperor asked, "If one is like a Taoist who knows how to preserve energy, might he be able to preserve the sex ability even until a hundred years of age?"

Chi'Po said, "Yes, A Taoist will be able to keep the sex ability and make a child even after a hundred years old."

The Yellow Emperor said, "Yes, I have heard about the Taoists. At an ancient time there were true men who recognized the order of the universe, who lived in accordance with yin yang principles and breathed the universal ki-energy. Since they were free from all troubles, they maintained vitality and their mind and body functioned harmoniously with Heaven and Earth so that their life was infinite.

"At the Middle Age there were supreme men who had the virtue of the order of the universe, lived according to yin yang principles and harmonized with the four seasons. They left this society and lived on a high mountain. They breathed good air and maintained perfect vitality. Therefore they could go anywhere they wished and know anything before it happened. These people are the true men. At the Recent Age there were virtuous men who lived in harmony with the four seasons and the day and night cycle and, therefore, never suffered from epidemic or bacterial diseases. They kept desire low, were never angry, and were not alienated from others. They didn't make their clothes too fashionable, did not overwork, kept the mind peaceful, and were satisfied with a simple life. They could have lived over a hundred years. At present there are wise men who imitate the life of the true men. However, they are not the true men. Therefore, they cannot live forever although they can extend their life because they live in accordance with the order of the universe and in harmony with seasonal changes.

"This is my understanding. I would like to be the true man so that I can rise to the heavens riding on a dragon."

Yin Syndrome

On March 25th my family went to San Francisco where Cornellia attended several private meetings. After the meetings we all went to see a movie – *China Syndrome*. It was a good, realistic, and humanistic movie – except the name. It should be called "Yin Syndrome" because the fear concerning nuclear radiation is one of the yin syndromes of modern civilization.

A few days later on the 28th, I was surprised to hear that the movie story became a reality at Three Mile Island. It was a timely accident, making a tremendous advertisement for the movie. A share in the Columbia Motion Picture Company went up almost five times, according to *Time*.

Due to the anti-nuclear movement by environmentalists, naturalists, health conscious faddists, etc., safety rules will be tighter and the cost of electricity will go up. This is Yin Syndrome Number One. Yin Syndrome Number Two is fear of nuclear radiation. Scientists are sure that large amounts of radiation are very dangerous. Exposure to 100 rems can result in radiation sickness which is characterized by anemia, hemorrhaging, and infection; 500 rems can be fatal. Most people absorb a total of about 200 millirems a year. About half of this (100 millirems) comes from natural background radioactivity. Such background radioactivity is blamed for an estimated 1 to 2 percent of all cancers. The remaining 100 millirems comes from man-made sources of radiation such as medical uses, wristwatches, microwave ovens, nuclear mining, and power-generating operations. However, it is widely debated as to what is the safe level of exposure to radiation. In recent years, several controversial studies suggest that there has been an increase in cancer caused by very low levels of radiation.

According to macrobiotic principles, radiation is yin and cancer is an extremely yin syndrome. Therefore, extreme radiation exposure will cause cancer. However, as Ohsawa said, there is no 'radiation sickness'. If we avoid the regular use of extremely yin foods such as sugar, alcohol, vinegar, coffee, tropical fruits, etc., we can immunize against yin radiation.

We don't need to be afraid of radiation. Fear of radiation is Yin Syndrome Number Two. According to statistics, Japan, who received the attack of two atomic bombs, is not the country with a high rate of leukemia; instead she is lowest. "All leukemia, childhood and adult, in modern countries is highest in Denmark (about 7.5), the United States (about 6.2), and Sweden (about 6.0). It is lowest in Japan (2.8), Portugal (3.3), and Iceland (4.7) (numbers per 100,000)." (From *The Savage Cell* by Pat McGrady, Basic Books, 1964.)

In conclusion, there are two types of yin syndromes. The first is psychological: nervousness, worry, passivity, introversion, spaced-out behavior, lack of concentration, lack of memory, slow decision-making. The second is physiological: acidity, anemia, hemorrhaging, swelling or reddening, protruding eyes, tiredness or lack of energy, slow movement, constipation (sometimes too yang), diarrhea, lack of appetite, leukemia, cancer, low blood pressure – in short, almost all modern sicknesses except certain heart diseases, skin diseases, constipation, etc.

The main cause of these yin syndromes is in our diet. By controlling our diet we can protect against yin syndromes and we can maintain a balanced, healthy and happy life.

The diet which causes yin syndromes in the temperate zone

is one which contains the following foods, consumed every day:

> Sugar and sugared foods
> Refined foods, especially grains
> Chemical additives, colorings
> Animal foods (especially grown with hormone feeds)
> Vinegar, spices, coffee
> Soft drinks, beer, wine, all other alcoholic drinks.

In the above list, the first three are the most important to eliminate in your diet. This will be the first step toward natural immunization against nuclear radiation.

Sagen Ishizuka

Sagen Ishizuka was born on February 4, 1851 at Fukui prefecture, two years before Admiral Perry arrived at Uraga Port asking to open trade between Japan and America.

He liked to study ever since he was young. He could understand Dutch, French, German, and English at age 18. Furthermore, his purpose in studying languages was not merely for the languages themselves. He studied in order to understand chemistry, medicine, and astronomy in those languages.

He had a skin disease by birth. When he was four years old, he suffered from prurigo over his whole body, and at age five he suffered from acute kidney disease. This kidney disease was the cause of his death at age fifty-nine. His skin disease was caused by the kidney disease, which in turn was caused by his mother who ate too much fish and spices during her pregnancy. This he learned later, through macrobiotic medicine and diet. He established a unique medicine from his studies of Oriental medicine.

At age twenty-eight, while he was on duty as an army doctor at Seinan Senso (the riot caused by T. Saigo, the famous army general of Kagoshima), this kidney disease caused severe swelling in his legs and eyelids, and protein secretions in the urine. At the age of thirty-two, he suffered from the severe kidney disease again. At that time he started to study the relationship of food to sickness (macrobiotic medicine and nutrition).

31

He tried to cure his sickness through Western medicine at first, or rather we can say that he was interested in studying medicine because of his desire to cure his chronic disease. After finding that Western medicine didn't make him any better, he started to study Oriental medicine. After studying both medicines, he finally found right foods to bring health to the Japanese. The *Nei Ching* says, "There are three categories of drugs, the lowest of which is poisonous; the second one is a little poisonous; the highest one is no poison. The lowest drug cures six out of ten sicknesses, leaving poisons in the patients. The middle one cures seven out of ten sicknesses, leaving a small amount of poison. Even the highest medicine can cure only eight or nine out of ten sicknesses. The sicknesses that medicine cannot cure can be cured only by foods."

Sagen reached the conclusion that foods are the highest medicine, after searching Western medicine for many years. He realized that all sickness and physical weakness is caused by wrong eating habits. In other words, he established a science of Foods for Health and Happiness. This is called *shokuyo* in Japanese, and was later called *macrobiotics* by George Ohsawa.

What is *shokuyo*? *Shoku* is all matter and energy which creates and nourishes the perfect man. *Yo* is the deed or way to nourish ourselves, with the knowledge of *shoku*. In other words, *shokuyo* is the right knowledge and proper deeds concerning creation and nourishment of the perfect healthy man.

The spirit or attitude of *shokuyo* medicine, which he applied to the sick, was entirely the opposite of that of Western medicine. He advised an azuki bean, brown rice diet for stomach disease, which a Western medical doctor would not dare to advise due to the belief that brown rice is hard to digest. He also advised burdock root, radish juice, brown rice, etc., which have no therapeutic value in modernized Japanese thought. He emphasized improved physical resistance against diseases, rather than curing sicknesses symptomatically.

Finally he reached the idea which divides all foods into two categories. One is the potassium category and the other is the sodium category. He explained not only sicknesses but also natural phenomena, such as seasonal changes and differentiation of living things, by potassium and sodium.

At the time of Ishizuka, nutritional theory was interested mostly in the three organic nutrients: protein, fat, and carbohydrate. In his opinion, the inorganic nutrients do compose most of the body; inorganic minerals control the functioning of the organs, metabolism, and the activities of the nervous system. According to Ishizuka, the most important inorganic minerals in our body are potassium (K) and sodium (Na). These two minerals have very similar characteristics, and it is difficult to distinguish one from the other. However, when they combine with acid and form salts, those salts are quite distinguishable. Potassium salts and sodium salts are antagonistic to each other in their function in the body – like the wife and husband in a family. Not only are they opposed to each other, they are complementary – as a wife relies on her husband and a husband relies on his wife. If we compare nutrients to the army, he said, carbohydrates are the soldiers which make up the majority of the army; proteins and fats are the officers; potassium is a general, while sodium is a lieutenant general.

Potassium salt activates oxidation and sodium salt inhibits oxidation. To illustrate this, add ash paste to a string and dry well. Tie a safety pin or paper clip to one end of the string, and hang the other end where it can hang freely. Then burn the string. The pin will fall down as the string burns. Next, add salt (NaCl) to a piece of string and dry it well. Follow the same procedure, hanging the string with the pin somewhere freely, and burn it. The string will burn up, but black ashes will keep the pin from falling, because the salt on the string prevents complete oxidation. The incomplete combustion makes black ashes.

Therefore, if one eats grains and vegetables, which contain much potassium, the blood will oxidize well and allow better physiological functioning. On the other hand, if one eats a lot of meats, poultry, fish, and eggs, which contain high amounts of sodium, blood oxidation is not so good, leaving much poisonous acid. Therefore, vegetarians live longer and eaters of animal food live a shorter life. Since the air near the ocean has more sodium than the air in the mountains, people who live near the ocean have shorter lives than people who live in the mountains.

Potassium salt catches fire and burns quickly, but also has the characteristic of reducing heat and keeping cool. Potassium salt has been used in medicine for heat reduction. If one applies ash paste over the skin, it keeps the skin cool. Contrary to K salt, Na salt burns slower and has the characteristic of increasing heat and keeping warm. For example, firewood grown far from the ocean catches fire easily and burns well; the ashes are white. In contrast, it is more difficult to start a fire with firewood grown at the oceanside, and the wood burns more slowly. The ashes are black.

The Japanese custom is to cremate a person who dies. If he has been vegetarian the ash will be white, but if he has been eating a lot of animal foods the ash will be black. Therefore, if a monk dies and his ash is black, he proves himself not to have been a very highly spiritual monk. If his ash is white, he is proven to have been a spiritual, honest monk.

Dr. Ishizuka discusses K salt and Na salt much more in his Japanese text, *Chemical Diet for Longevity* (Haku Bunkan, 1896). He claims that physiological differences (such as color of the skin, fat or thin, big or small, speed of growth, strength, longevity, sickness, voice, good or bad memory, etc.) are all dependent on environmental conditions and the intake of K salt and Na salt foods. Dr. Ishizuka applied this K salt and Na salt relationship to his patients. He advised eating more K salt type foods if the symptoms are Na type. If the patient had a K salt type sickness, he advised eating Na type foods.

After his book was published, he was so famous that he had to consult one hundred patients every day. His treatment used no medicines, but dietary suggestions exclusively. People thought the diet he recommended was outdated. However, his advice cured so many people that he became more and more famous. Letters from patients could reach him addressed merely: "Tokyo, Dr. Anti-Doctor."

After his death, his disciples established the *Shoku-Yo-Kai Macrobiotic Association*. When this association was almost bankrupt, a young man who had cured his many sicknesses by the brown rice diet of Dr. Ishizuka worked hard, putting his money to reorganize the Association. The Association became famous again and hundreds of patients came every day. This young man was George Ohsawa. He was not only good at business, but he also studied hard on Ishizuka's theory.

When Ohsawa learned Ishizuka's theory, he realized that a concept which explained the relationship between the two salts of K and Na had existed in the Orient for thousands of years. After several years of study, he changed Ishizuka's K salt and Na salt to the terminology of yin and yang.

Printing and Tempura

There is a common principle between offset printing and tempura cooking.

Water is one of the most interesting, useful, and important substances in the universe. We know without water there is no life. Biologically speaking, water is the source of life. Chemically speaking, water is a solvent. Water dissolves everything into parts. It dissolves even the atom into ionized conditions. (A positive ion is an atomic condition in which an atom loses an electron; a negative ion is a condition in which it gains an electron.) From its dissolving and dividing characteristic, we classify water as yin.

Physically speaking, however, water is yang. It travels in a downward direction, which is yang, from higher to lower places, such as in streams, creeks, and rivers. Rivers never run from ocean to mountain. Rain always comes from above. Further, water is very yang physically because it is indestructible. This is an amazing characteristic. Even under a million tons of pressure, water (all liquids) will never break. Therefore, water is used for hydraulic pressure.

Even though water has such yang qualities, macrobiotics considers that because it opposes fire and cools off heat, water is yin. It absorbs much heat. For this reason, the temperature near the ocean stays about the same day and night but inland temperatures change drastically from day to night. If we had

36

enough water, we could extinguish the fire of the sun. Couldn't we? How much water would it take? Please calculate, if you like mathematics.

Being liquid, oil has characteristics similar to water. It also is indestructible. We use oil as a lubricant, changing it from time to time – not because it breaks down but because it becomes dirty. This is the yang character of oil. However, we consider oil yin. Why? Oil is a solvent (it dissolves some substances). Oil is lighter than water. Oil makes a thin film. But the most important reasoning that oil is yin lies in the fact that oil and water dislike, or repel, each other. Therefore if water is yin, oil must also be yin, because yin and yin repel each other. This repelling characteristic of oil and water has been used both in the printing industry and in Oriental cooking.

This page is printed by offset printing. Offset printing is the process of creating a printed image from a flat plate on which an image has been photographically imposed. The plate itself is receptive to water; therefore, it rejects ink. The material used in creating the image is receptive to the oil-based ink, which rejects water. The inked image is transferred onto a rubber-covered cylinder which then transfers it to the paper. If the cylinder which is covered by the plate is given water, the surface will be covered with water except images which reject water. Then ink is given to the rollers, which transfer ink to the images.

In tempura cooking, oil is heated up. After it reaches a high temperature, sliced and battered vegetables are dropped in. This method of cooking is called tempura. Since it creates very delicious and beautiful dishes, almost all Japanese restaurants serve tempura. According to Ohsawa, tempura is one of the most yangizing forms of cooking. Why? What is the mechanism of tempura cooking? This style is an application of the fact that oil and water do not mix with each other. When battered vegetables are dropped into hot oil, oil coats the surface of the vegetables. The water in the batter and in the vegetables heats up and becomes steam. However, the surrounding oil prevents the steam from evaporating. Therefore, the pressure goes up and the temperature goes up too. Tempura cooks vegetables without allowing them to lose their own water, and this means their own nutrients as well. This is the reason that foods, especially vegetables, cooked by the tempura method are so delicious.

The above two processes are some of the applications of yin and yin. You can create more applications with yin and yin, as well as yin and yang or yang and yang. Please apply the principle of yin and yang to your life, and be creative.

April 1980

The Story of Soba

It is recorded that soba was already being eaten around 710 in Japan. At that time soba was not a noodle, but shaped like a tortilla. It was eaten after being roasted on a fire. Then *soba-gaki* was developed. Buckwheat flour was mixed with hot water and eaten with sauce. It was around 1700 when soba noodles started to appear among people's dishes. Strangely enough, soba noodles were customarily served at the restaurants in one bowl only. One could not order seconds Of course, the noodles were made by hand.

It is commonly believed that soba is best produced around Kurohime Mountain in Nagano-ken. One theory says that the county named Sarashina in Nagano-ken was named thus because someone planted buckwheat seeds in this area brought from the Saracen Empire (Middle East). From this legend, Sarashina soba is the most famous brand name of soba noodles in Japan.

In the beginning, soba noodles were served simply in three forms: *mori* (noodles served separately with a sauce on the side); *kake* (noodles served in a soup); and *soba-gaki* (mentioned above). However, about a hundred years ago the port of Nagasaki opened and European and Chinese dishes were introduced. Many people started to eat new dishes. As a result, soba restaurants became less popular. In order to increase customers, new kinds of dishes were invented, adding fishcake, egg, chicken meat, mushrooms, *fu* (wheat gluten), *yuba* (soymilk 'crepe'), and vegetables to the top of the noodles. Some of those noodle dishes are called by the following names:

Tempura Soba – Vegetable or shrimp tempura topped over the noodles, served in *kake* style. This is very popular among foreigners.

Yamakake soba – Noodles topped with grated *yama-imo* (a cultivated *jinenjo-imo*, a most yang radish-shaped potato). This is served in *kake* style.

Tsukimi soba – Over easy egg on top of the noodles. Served in *kake* style.

Ankake soba – Noodles topped by kuzu sauce and served in *kake* style.

Mori soba with *yama-imo* – Noodles eaten and dipped into the grated *yama-imo* sauce served *mori* style.

Mori soba with grated radish – When I was in Boston several years ago, I visited Mr. Hayashi, chef of the Seventh Inn. It was almost midnight, so he served us an instant soba which was the most delicious soba I ever ate. It requires very little cooking, so you can serve it for unexpected guests you wish to treat nicely. Boil soba noodles, drain, and serve with grated *daikon* radish, natural soy sauce, green scallions, and *nori*.

Kaki tama soba [or *Tanuki* (badger) *soba*] – A soup is made using small pieces of deep-fried batter which are saved during tempura cooking. This is an inexpensive, quick way to make noodle soup. Noodles are served with this soup in *kake* style.

(Note: In legend, the badger had the power to deceive people, and this mock tempura soup is also deceptive.)

Tori-Nanban soba – Noodles are topped with chicken and sliced scallion in *kake* style.

Kitsune soba – According to legend, *kitsune* is a fox who likes fried tofu (*age*). Therefore, this is a soba noodle dish topped with *age* and served in *kake* style.

There are many more soba dishes.

Buckwheat is a very yang grain; it is probably the most yang grain. Therefore, soba noodles are served in a colder climate – that is to say, the northern part of Japan. Soba restaurants existed only in Tokyo or north of Tokyo. By the same token, wheat noodles (called udon) are yin. Udon was eaten in southern Japan and udon restaurants existed only in southern Japan in places such as Kyoto, Osaka, and Kyushu. Today there is no longer such a distinction; you can eat soba in the south and udon in the north. However, in the north the noodle shop is still called *Soba-ya*, and in the south it is called *Udon-ya*.

If you live in a very cold place, or you have a very yin constitution, soba (buckwheat) may be better than rice. On the contrary, if you live in a warmer climate or you have a very yang constitution, eat wheat noodles more often.

Mr. Makoto Kano, who pioneered Kurohime Enmei Cha (herb tea company) and a natural living commune in Japan after World War II, had been eating soba every day for over twenty years, because soba was the only food available there. As a result, he became so yang, he doesn't even go near soba restaurants. He simply cannot even smell soba!

April 1980

Appreciation

When illness is cured, we tend to forget how much we appreciated the medicine that relieved the pain. It seems to me the same thing happens in macrobiotics. For a while after the pains are gone or troubles are solved by macrobiotics, we tend to forget its value. When we forget the value of macrobiotics, we also forget to show appreciation toward the works and inspirations of George Ohsawa.

It is difficult to appreciate someone's works and teachings when we never saw him. Newcomers to macrobiotics never met Ohsawa, so it may be natural that they are not much appreciative of him and his works. I feel this kind of macrobiotic practice lacks deep roots and will die out sooner or later. Without Ohsawa, macrobiotics would never have existed in the world as it is today.

Ohsawa taught us that appreciation is the foundation of happiness and the macrobiotic way of life. I agree with him. There are at least six categories of appreciation.

1. Appreciation to natural resources including air, water, foods, and gasoline.

2. Appreciation to society which supplies our needs.

3. Appreciation for our ancestors and parents, who made our life possible.

4. Appreciation to our mate, who makes our life most beautiful and difficult.

5. Appreciation to our teachers and friends who teach us how to live a happy life as well as give us severe scoldings and criticism.

6. Appreciation to ourselves who are creating a beautiful life, have faith in the natural order, and don't give up in the face of difficulties.

July 1980

Five American Girls
European Lecture Tour

At the beginning of 1979 I started plans to go to Europe to give lectures and cooking classes. Later, when Cornellia and I went to Japan with Bob and Betty Kennedy, we met with Clim Yoshimi and Francoise Riviere in Tokyo and took a trip to Kyoto and Osaka together. At that time Cornellia promised Clim that we would be at his center in Paris the next May to help out his center's promotion. As soon as I returned to America in October I started to arrange the European trip. I worried that we couldn't help his center much; rather that he would help us instead. This trip ended up more or less the opposite of what I expected. I failed where I expected to succeed, and I succeeded where I didn't expect.

The places I visited in Europe during November of 1978 were rather less exciting but at the places we visited this time we experienced overwhelming excitement and welcome. This excitement and welcome was mostly due to five American girls who married European boys and started operating macrobiotic centers there. Without these five girls, my lecture trip would not have been successful.

The first one we met was Barbara Berger Gertsen, who married Tue Gertsen about ten years ago in Copenhagen. They started a macrobiotic center there. Barbara never learned macrobiotics from any teacher personally; she learned everything from books – even cooking. Cornellia's cooking class was

44

the first one she ever attended. So you can imagine what kind of macrobiotic meals she cooked at the beginning. Her uniqueness is not only that. She was educated at a very exclusive Ivy League girls school in New York. Her father was a high officer at the Pentagon who directed the Vietnam War, and she was a pacifist opposed to the war. She married a conscientious objector. Her mother was a professional golfer who never cooked at home.

She ran away from home at nineteen, quit school, fled to the slums of New York City and lived on the Lower East Side. She became involved in the artistic, intellectual, and political underground and was influenced by Camus, Bob Dylan, marijuana, hashish, LSD, the New Left, etc., etc. Then she travelled with her first husband to Holland, Belgium, France, Italy, Israel, Spain, New York City again, England, New York again, Canada, back to New York, and then to Mexico. She was almost dying when she arrived in Mexico where she met a famous Swedish painter, Ragnar Johansson, who invited them to come to Sweden.

She wrote her experiences in a book form and published it in 1967. It is a crazy and very unhappy book. It is full of doubt, misery, and frustration. She wrote, "Shall i light a fuse to this bomb that i am? i/time bomb/and blow up, explode out into the world universe in a fullness of force/time bomb/me, give up everything for this explosion that moment which will be existence on the level of pure energy?" Now, she is the mother of three children, a good teacher of macrobiotics in a country with the highest rate of abortion in the world. Her second macrobiotic book, *Reflections of a Macrobiotic Housewife,* is one of the macrobiotic bestsellers in Europe. She changed herself completely from unhappiness to happiness.

The most amazing thing about her is that she doesn't seem to care about the living conditions of her home. Her living conditions at present cannot be comfortable for a girl like her who grew up in the middle-class family of a U.S. government official. She is the only American girl I met who never went home during her marriage, living far away from home. She was too poor and busy, like our life was when we lived in New York. Most American girls will not dare to make such a sacrifice. She seems to have no trouble sacrificing her life. No, she has no sacrifice because she is doing what she really wants to do. In her dictionary there is no such word as sacrifice. She is a rare woman, even in an Erehwon. What made our trip most meaningful was meeting with her and Tue. For this I give my most sincere thanks to them.

In Belgium, Marc Van Cauwenberghe gave me a four-thousand-page collection of all of Ohsawa's writings (translations in French and English) which have not been published yet in book form although many of them have been published in various magazines. This collection is the result of over ten years of constant research, interest, and appreciation of George Ohsawa and his work. I sincerely appreciate his effort and his work. I promised him that G.O.M.F. will publish this in book form.

A girl who was sitting next to Marc gave me unyielding opinion against my lecture when I was talking about the Order of Man but not the universe. It turned out she was Marc's wife, an American girl who is distinguished from European girls by giving her opinions freely. She is very yang and has an American spirit. She will be a good combination with Marc, who is a scientist and rather introverted type of person. She will make Marc's life very interesting.

The next American girl I met was not really American but a Korean girl. Sook is the wife of Rob de Nies of Hasselt, Belgium and is also very yang. Rob was in San Francisco two years ago and had a good time; at that time I met him when I lectured at Fort Mason. I even ate his lunch, served at the lecture time. I didn't meet Sook at that time, so she was waiting for Cornellia and me to come to Hasselt, a small town located in the eastern part of Belgium, close to Germany. Macrobiotics has been growing very rapidly around here because one boy cured his multiple sclerosis by the macrobiotic diet. Egidius Musiek started a food store and restaurant here two years ago. It was too busy, so the food store and restaurant were separated. In the restaurant, Rob is helping Egidius, and other members of the center are working at the food store. In my opinion, the yang character of Sook will be the energy supporting Rob and this community in the yin Belgian climate.

When we arrived at Lausanne it was already past midnight. I was afraid nobody would pick us up at the Swiss station because my train was changed to the summer schedule and I was not sure whether or not a French friend confirmed our arrival time with Mario and Marlise in Lausanne. I was relieved when we saw a tall couple approach us with a bunch of flowers at the midnight station. It was Mario and Marlise Binetti.

I learned later that I had told Mario at the French Meadows Summer Camp that he would marry soon. After summer camp he went back to Texas where he was studying at the University, and married Marlise. After the marriage they moved to Lausanne because Switzerland is Mario's native country. Eighteen months ago they began helping Paul Simon, who started the macrobiotic center here. This center occupies two buildings. Lectures, food sales, and business offices are in one building, and a restaurant is in another. Their last summer camp was very successful, attended by 300 people per day. The center is much developed considering the fact that it was started only three years ago. The only shortcoming of this center is the lack of a leader. In this chaotic situation, the presence of a tough American girl will be a good balance. Being the daughter of a pioneer, Marlise will be a macrobiotic pioneer on another continent.

The last American girl I met was Kim Bradford, who is also a pioneer girl. She is living in London, not Switzerland, and comes from California, not Texas. Peter Bradford is one of the founders of Sunwheel, a macrobiotic importing, wholesale, and restaurant business in London. I forgot to ask how Peter married Kim. However, Kim is the exact same type as Marlise, and Peter is the same as Mario. Peter is doing a job similar to Mario's in Lausanne, and shows similar character. Kim is helping Peter like Marlise is helping Mario. Kim will be a great help because of her good American-style nature.

The only shortcoming of these three girls out of the five is that they are too sentimental. They have to visit America too often. This is their sentimentality. I very much appreciate their help with our trip. I also hope for the development of their judgment. Through this they will acquire real happiness.

Reflections on My Accident

Cornellia and I flew to St. Louis, Missouri by prearranged flight on June 13th from Sacramento. From Sacramento to Denver there is a one-hour time difference, and another hour difference exists between Denver and St. Louis. The total flying time was about four hours but counting the time difference we were in the air six hours. Therefore, two meals were served – breakfast between Sacramento and Denver, and lunch between Denver and St. Louis. I was so greedy, I ate all meals including meat sausages; however, I didn't touch the sugary cake. These meals caused headaches for two days.

At St. Louis, two Toms were awaiting us. One was a miso-making Tom from Massachusetts who had been in the Ohio Miso Company. He told us he left that company and is starting another miso company in Massachusetts.

It took about three hours from St. Louis to the campsite at Moniteau Farm where I stopped over last summer on our lecture trip. When we visited then, the Farm had just begun the property sale; now, almost all properties have been sold except one parcel. They said about fifty people are living here including many children.

Bill and Dale and their wives started the summer camp at Bowling Green, Missouri; Cornellia and I attended and gave lectures two years ago. They couldn't make the summer camp last year because they had just moved here. This time the camp was much different than that of two years ago. The land is owned by them. About four hundred acres of land has been divided into about thirty sections. This kind of ownership or sales is impossible in California, according to my experience; I tried to make a macrobiotic community near Chico about eight years ago but failed because of too many state restrictions on land development and division.

It was about 7:00 when we arrived at the camp. We met familiar faces: Bill, Dale, Rita, Sandy, Jean (Tom's wife – I knew her from San Francisco times), Pat and Meredith McCarty, and Bill Tims were there. Dinner was served for us, and the chef was our old friend Loren who was as joyous as ever. There were a few more people I knew. After talking with them for a while, we went to bed. I was tired.

The next day (Saturday, June 14), the camp started. I gave lectures three mornings, followed by Cornellia's cooking and child care classes. There were lectures by Jerome, Bill, Pat, and Jean Kohler. Their lectures were all very interesting. One night Dr. Kohler gave a piano concert at the old barn house. I never heard a piano concert in a barn. People were listening all over the place – on chairs, on the ground, on the floor, and on the hay. It was a good performance.

On the night of the 18th, they organized a talent show. I was surprised the show was so well organized. I enjoyed it very much. When the party was over, I asked Dale who would be driving us to the airport the next morning. He introduced me to another Tom who had taken pictures of my lectures and presented me. I made sure we should start leaving at 5:00 a.m.

On Thursday, June 19th, Cornellia and I got up at 4:00 a.m., packed our stuff, and waited for Tom outside the tent around 4:30. Around 5:00, one pickup passed by the tent and passed by again a few moments later. Then there was no sound and no light. We started to worry. I went to see if there were any signs of a car moving around Jerome's tent because his car was to be used that morning. Cornellia was irritated and she asked me to stay around the tent and not walk.

Around 5:15, one van came to the tent. The second Tom was driving. He said the car was found but not the key, so he borrowed the van; however, he didn't know whose van it was. It was becoming late, so we started, along with Tom's girl-friend. After driving five minutes, Tom realized he forgot a check which was Spiral Inn's payment for G.O.M.F. books, and also some miso koji Cornellia bought from Spiral Inn. He asked me whether he must drive back to pick up those things or not. I said yes. So the van went back to where his truck was parked. When we arrived there, I noticed that it was Jean's property. Therefore, the van must be hers. Cornellia said Jacques's tent was there, pointing towards the woods to the north. I said his tent was further east, after the bridge. Since she continued to persuade her opinion and I knew Jacques's tent was far, I shouted, "Are you crazy?" This upset the feelings of Cornellia and maybe the feelings of Tom.

When we started to drive again it was already 5:30. The sun was not up yet but the darkness of night was fading away. It was becoming lighter. After we passed Jamestown, I must have slept. I awoke when I heard someone try to help me up. I was lying on the floor on my stomach. I couldn't move. I realized we had had an accident. I saw Cornellia and Tom's girlfriend. They were shocked but they could move. I couldn't move.

Awhile later Tom came back after telephoning Spiral Inn. He was hardly injured at all. Cornellia told me the car turned over once and finally rolled into a ditch. All windows were broken except the windshield glass. Tom said the van rolled twice after slipping on the wet downgrade curve. He lost control because the car vibrated heavily at the rear. When he braked, the car rolled, I thought. Anyway, we were lucky because the van stood on four wheels after rolling into the ditch. Tom said he wasn't hurt, except for a few scratches, because he was holding onto the steering wheel. Cornellia said her handbag and the miso koji box were thrown out, far away, and she had to pick them up. She also said we were lucky that no one was thrown from the car. If we had been thrown out, we would be severely injured or dead.

A while later Sandy came with her van. Two helped me up from the ditch and then to the van. I couldn't move, but I had no pain. At Spiral Inn, Robert let me stay in his mobile home in order to lie down and receive tofu plasters. Tofu was brought from a nearby town, and Cornellia applied it to my shoulder and back. She changed them every three or four hours.

Since our tickets were invalid, Bill said we had to see a doctor who could give an accident certificate to the airline so that they would extend our tickets. We asked the doctor to come, but Bill said he would not. Cornellia wanted to go back home on the 20th (the next day), so we arranged to go to the doctor's office the next day, get the paper, and go to the airport.

Rita came and checked my blood pressure. It was 160/90. I had a good appetite. I ate two times on the 19th and also on the 20th. I drank tea with a spoon. Hugh gave me a tamari serving bottle with tea. I could drink tea at any time. Problems were urination and bowel movement. I tried urination in bed in vain. So I had no urination or bowel movement on the 19th.

When night came I self-reflected: why did I have an accident? Ohsawa said a macrobiotic person never has an accident. I must have done something wrong. I recalled what happened in the morning. My shouting. I did this because I wanted Cornellia to be more gentle and listen to others' opinions. I did the same thing last year. When she caused an accident last year, I wrote an article saying she had an accident because she didn't listen to my critiques. I wanted to teach Cornellia to be a good student rather than a teacher. I was not giving her kind consideration; I knew she fell asleep driving because she did not have enough sleep during preparations for summer camp. I was cold. I should not have blamed her in such a way. I advised her to be a student, making myself a teacher. I tried to change her character. It was my arrogance, I thought. Therefore, I had an accident. I can't change her. Nobody can change her except herself. I will accept her as she is.

As my thoughts reached like this, my mind became very peaceful. I thought I found the cause of the accident, and I slept.

The next morning (Friday the 20th) there was no pain but I couldn't get up. The plan was changed. Bill asked the doctor to come. Bill told us he would come the next day. There was no pain as long as I lay on my back. I couldn't move. I kept my face toward the right, which made me painless. The most pain came when I coughed. When mucus came up and choked the bronchial tubes or windpipe, then I coughed and had the most pain. So whenever coughing, I tried not to cough unconsciously. I drank a little tea which was successful sometimes. If it was not successful and mucus blocked the windpipe or bronchial tubes, then I was miserable.

I realized my breathing was shallow. I was not breathing from the abdomen. My abdominal muscle was tight. Hugh gave me an abdominal massage to try and relieve tension in my breathing center (near the belly-button - probably *kiketsu* of the kidney meridian). It made my breathing easier.

Hugh introduced me to David Wilson who is a medical doctor and has been macrobiotic after he suffered a cancer. He told me I may have broken one or two ribs, and that might be the reason my abdomen was so tight and breathing difficult.

Finally I managed to urinate in the bed. I was so happy. When I was healthy, urination was a daily routine work. I gave no attention to it. Now I could not get up, and urination was a major job. I appreciated so much that I could urinate.

That night I had a funny dream. I was in a big field which was full of strange plastic stuff – all car parts. They gradually moved in circles. I never saw such things. Then what is dreaming? I was seeing what I had never seen before. What I saw was all illusion. I wondered if I may have injured my brain.

The next morning (21st) I could move my neck more, so I kept my head straight. Then gradually breathing became difficult. Hugh and David came to see me. When I was talking with them, my breathing was choked. I could hardly breathe. It was harder and harder. In the afternoon a doctor came to inspect my condition. My condition was the worst – I was almost dying. I couldn't breathe. He insisted on taking an x-ray right away. I told him I would wait until Monday. I was choked. I was moaning. No one knew what happened. Cornellia worried. She prayed to God for my easement. I was choked, choked, and choked. Hard breathing had been continuous from 9:00 in the morning until 3:00 in the afternoon.

Cornellia apologized for being so stubborn. I was already accepting her stubbornness, so I said, "That is not your fault." She cried and I cried. Then all of a sudden I realized the real cause of the accident.

The real cause of my accident was forgetting my promise to God. I promised God that I would observe the number seven diet and give prayers on the 18th and 24th of every month in order to appreciate George Ohsawa and his teachings; however, I had forgotten my promise completely. I didn't do any number seven diet or give prayer. I even went fishing instead. My accident is the result of breaking my commitment. I understood clearly why I had an accident. As soon as I had this reflection, I remembered the Sotai teaching which advises us to always find a body position that makes us feel good. However, I could only move my head, so I moved my head toward the right. What a miracle – my hard breathing and choking stopped. My breathing returned to that of yesterday. Until

Friday I had pain in the left shoulder, so my head faced right. However, Saturday morning I had less pain in the shoulder, so I had been talking with people facing straight and lying straight. This position must have choked my windpipe or bronchial tubes. What a simple movement to make such a big difference. I appreciated the teaching of Sotai which saved my life – at least my acute choking.

After my breathing returned to normal again, I decided to go back home. Hugh found an airline flying direct from St. Louis to San Francisco instead of changing at Denver. He contacted his family so they would meet us at the San Francisco airport and drive us to Sacramento where we could pick up our car at the airport parking lot.

On Sunday the 22nd I was breathing normally. It was like a nightmare that I had severe choking yesterday. After the second tofu plaster change on my shoulder and back, Hugh and David came and bandaged my left side ribs. I was able to slowly lift my upper body; I could even sit on a chair. Lying on my back for four days made me weak, but I could even walk. In the evening Tom drove his car next to the mobile home. Helped by two, I slowly moved to his car. I managed to sit in the front seat. I had no pain. Wonderful. Finally, I could go back home. As Tom drove, I sat in the front seat. I was very comfortable. I appreciated the good job done by David and Hugh; without their help I don't know how I could get back. At St. Louis, Tom offered us to stay at his apartment. It was a very hot night. I couldn't lie down, so I sat and slept in that position on the bed.

On Monday the 23rd Tom took us to the airport. There I was given a wheelchair and the airline company let us board first. There were no difficulties boarding and disembarking, as I had worried before. My bandage was working perfectly. I could even write this memoir on the flight, as well as read books. Cornellia brought rice balls on board. I ate them instead of the flight meal this time. The flight arrived in San Francisco on time.

We met with Betsy and her two sons at the airport. They came from Sacramento to pick us up. I appreciated this kindness very much. Hugh and later Betsy drove their wagon bus. It was around 5:00 p.m. when we arrived at the Sacramento airport, where we had a picnic prepared by Betsy.

Then we changed to my car which had been parked there just eleven days. The battery was dead because the water was evaporated by strong sun for eleven days. We added water and made a quick charge at the nearest station. It worked. Betsy drove her bus home, and Hugh drove us in our car to our home in Oroville.

We arrived home around 8:00 p.m. Hugh took the bandage off. I had hard breathing, so I sat instead of lying down. As long as my head was high I could breathe easily. Therefore, he recommended that Cornellia get a mechanical bed which can be adjusted for the head.

On Tuesday the 24th, Carl and Sandy got me a bed from Chico. That was a big help; that was the only thing I needed. Using this, I could get on the bed or get out of bed to go to the bathroom by myself easily.

At home, Cornellia and I shaved our heads and applied tofu plasters to protect from possible brain hemorrhage. I did this for a week. Cornellia gave me tofu plasters until the following Monday. Sometimes she applied rice plasters which worked very well on the shoulder.

I became better every day. I could move my head and waist a little more each day. I could drive the car on July 9, twenty days after the accident.

October 1980

Curing Cancer Is Not Enough

I

I recently read Norman Cousins's article in the June 1980 issue of the *Saturday Review*, "Being Healthy Is Not Enough." In this, Cousins said the death rate from heart disease for all ages has dropped 22 percent since 1968. I couldn't believe this, so I checked the statistic of the death rate in the U.S.A. in *Vital Statistics of the U.S.*, published by the government in 1980. To my amazement, the death rate from heart disease dropped 10 percent during 1960-1977, and cardiovascular disease dropped 16 percent in the same period. Is this a sign that the American health condition is improving? Norman Cousins checked the statistics further and he found that accidents and murders are replacing heart disease.

Similarly, I couldn't believe that the health of Americans is improving, so I investigated the statistics further. I found that cancer is replacing cardiovascular disease. In other words, the cancer death rate increased 16 percent during the period of 1960 to 1977.

Statistically, Americans changed their cause of death from cardiovascular disease to cancer. And the death by cancer seems to be increasing. What does this mean?

Heart and cardiovascular diseases kill us suddenly, almost without notice. It manifests a yang (contractive) symptom;

therefore it must be the result of the overconsumption of extreme yang foods such as beef, chicken, fish, pork, cheese, and so on.

On the contrary, cancer manifests very gradually. Cancer patients usually don't know they have cancer at the early stage. In most cases, by the time they have recognized their cancer it is too late. Therefore, cancer is a very yin (expansive) disease and it must be the result of the overconsumption of extreme yin substances such as sugar, alcohol, and chemicals.

There is another difference between heart disease and cancer. Heart disease is a disease of blood and muscle, while cancer is a disease of cells. This is one reason cancer is difficult to cure. Since modern medicine doesn't understand cell growth, it is obvious that medicine does not know how to cure abnormal growth. Arthur Guyton states in his textbook *Function of the Human Body* (4th Edition, W. B. Saunders Co., 1974, p. 41): "In the normal human body, regulation of cell growth and reproduction is mainly a mystery. We know almost nothing about the mechanisms that maintain proper numbers of the different types of cells in the body."

Why is it that modern medicine cannot understand the regulation of cell growth, the mechanism of growth? In my opinion, the reason is that modern medicine has misunderstood the origin of cells as well as the origin of cancer cells.

Dr. K. Morishita states in his small pamphlet *The Hidden Truth of Cancer* (G.O.M.F., 1976, p. 17), "The belief in Virchow's concept that 'a cell comes only from another cell' is the major obstacle to a study of the true origin of the cancer cell. If this theory is true, a cancer cell must come from another cancer cell. As a result of this thinking, three theories have been proposed concerning the origin of cancer cells: 1. A cancer cell has been introduced from the outside... 2. A cancer cell has existed in the body from the embryonic stage... 3. The sudden mutation of normal cells to cancer cells."

According to modern medicine, the first two have not received much support, and the last idea is the most accepted. Therefore, scientists are looking for the agents which cause this mutation; as a result, they have found thousands of carcinogens and other possible causes of cancer. The following are the major causes of cancer according to modern medicine:

Carcinogens: coal tar, color dyes, estrogen, arsenic, asbestos, etc.

Radiation

Smoking

Viruses

Warburg theory: Normal cells change to cancer cells by insufficient oxygen supply

Stress theory: Normal cells change to cancer cells by emotions such as worry, resentment, anger, etc.

The latter is not always the case; sometimes even peaceful, loving persons have cancer. Several years ago Rev. Suzuki roshi, founder of the San Francisco Zen Center, died from cancer. He kept a peaceful, loving mind all the way to death. In 1979, a famous Japanese magazine, *Bungei Shunju*, contained an article on the attitudes of fifty persons who suffered and died from cancer. The stories revealed the most amazingly peaceful and loving mentality that cancer patients can have.

Contrary to the above modern medical view, Doctors K. Chishima and K. Morishita think that cells are formed from blood. "Cells are formed from organic matter which has no constitution of cells. Nucleus and DNA are produced from protein." (*Cause, Prevention and Cure of Cancer*, K. Chishima, Neo-Haematology Society Press, Japan, p. 8.)

In my opinion, cancer cells might be produced either from normal cells or blood – which are of course produced from the foods we eat. Our food is the origin of cells. Without food,

there are no cells. Without food, there are no germ cells or
soma cells. Foods produce cancer cells. Foods cause the mutation of normal cells to cancer cells. Without this understanding
there will be no cure of cancer, as seen in the statistics.

How, then, does food produce cancer cells or mutations?
Our body cells are living in the body fluid which is always kept
alkaline, as Alexis Carrel said. "The intraorganic medium
never becomes acid. This fact is all the more surprising as
tissues unceasingly produce large quantities of carbonic, lactic,
sulphuric acids, etc., which are set free into the lymph. These
acids do not modify the reaction of blood plasma, because they
are neutralized, or rather buffered, by the presence of bicarbo-
nates and phosphates." (*Man, The Unknown*, Harper & Row,
1961.)

Our body maintains an alkalinity of body fluids not only by
its buffer system, but also by the foods we eat. There are two
kinds of foods. One is acid forming and the other is alkaline
forming. If one eats more acid forming than alkaline forming
foods for a long time, the body fluid will increase its acidity
and reach an almost acidic condition – that is to say, a pH of
less than 7.0.

When the body fluid reaches pH 6.9, coma results. Therefore, if the body fluid measures between pH 7.0 and 6.9, cells
try to live in this environment. Some will die, and some may
adapt in this environment. This adaptation will be the result of
the transmutation of genes. By the new genes, cells can live in
the acidic condition and without oxygen. This is the birth of
cancer cells. The cancer cell can live in the worst condition of
body fluids – that is to say, acidic fluid.

Therefore, in my opinion, cancer is a result of body adaptability and the body's final effort to survive in the polluted
internal environment (acidic body fluid). Therefore, cancer
cells can feed on normal cells' waste, which will be abundant in
our body. In other words, once normal cells change to cancer

cells or cancer cells are produced from blood, the cancer cells can live indefinitely until normal cells die. (Of course, if cancer cells outgrow the normal cells of a certain organ, then the organ ceases normal function and death eventually results.) This is the reason cancer cure is difficult. If a cancer cell once grows, it is almost impossible to change it back to a normal cell because it feeds on the waste products of normal cells which are always present in our body as long as we live.

Therefore, once a cancer cell grows, the only thing we can hope to do is to stop further growth. In order to do this we have to avoid eating strong acid forming foods such as sugar, alcohol, beef, chicken, pork, fish, eggs, and cheese. Although fruits are alkaline forming foods, fruits should be avoided by cancer patients because fruits contain lots of disaccharides which promote the growth of cancer cells. Cancer patients must observe a diet which consists of whole grains, beans, all vegetables (except very yin ones such as potato, eggplant, and tomato), seaweeds, seeds; natural alkaline condiments such as miso, soy sauce, and sea salt; and natural herb teas, such as twig tea. They must avoid all animal foods (including eggs, cheese, milk, milk products) and chemicalized, processed foods such as foods with coloring or preservatives added, etc.

In short, cancer patients must observe a strict form of the macrobiotic diet.

Then, is this enough to cure cancer?

II

I had a friend who had cancer without knowing it. When he met Ohsawa, he started macrobiotics very faithfully. He studied macrobiotics very well from Ohsawa. Ohsawa was a spiritual father, a guru for him. He became a leader of macrobiotics, giving lectures and publishing a magazine. He was so strongly attached to Ohsawa, he almost lost his mind when Ohsawa died in 1966. Then, according to his wife, he started eating out often at regular restaurants and drinking coffee. Then his cancer started growing again. In 1967, he was so sick that he went to Japan to get treatment for his cancer, but it was too late and he died in Japan. The autopsy revealed that he had had a cancer many years ago. In other words, his seven years of macrobiotics didn't cure it, but stopped its growth.

Another friend of mine had cancer when he was in Japan. Then he met Ohsawa and started the diet. This apparently stopped his cancer, but he thought the cancer was cured. Then he moved to America and started a macrobiotic restaurant. When this restaurant was established, he started a tour guide business for Japanese tourists. He often ate out with Japanese tourists at fancy restaurants where foods served were full of additives, chemicals, and colorings such as in animal foods.

He followed the macrobiotic principles over twenty years and his cancer must have been very small if not stopped. However, the cancer started to grow again. Within a year, he went to Japan for an operation and died there.

Mr. Ohmori, a cancer healer in Japan, once said that most cancer patients didn't live more than five years after they were cured with the macrobiotic diet. In my opinion, the cancer is not cured but just stopped from growing further; however, cancer can be kept under control as long as the macrobiotic diet is observed. This is not proof that macrobiotics is a temporary cure of less than five years, but rather it is proof, as Ohsawa often said, that macrobiotics is a 'once in a life' cure.

In order to cure cancer completely, one should deeply understand the order of the infinite universe – justice – so that he will observe the macrobiotic diet with true faith and pleasure, rather than just trying to cure symptomatically. This way he can live with the macrobiotic principles his whole life. With this understanding, he will inevitably change his lifestyle or diet sooner or later; without it, there will be no cure for cancer.

The understanding of the order of the infinite universe is what Ohsawa called faith. Without this faith, there is no curing of cancer. Cancer is a trial for man in order for him to reestablish faith in the order of the infinite universe. Without this faith, even a macrobiotic cure will be a temporal cure. In *Zen Macrobiotics* (Ohsawa Foundation, 1965, pp. 22-23), Ohsawa wrote:

> If you have faith, nothing shall be impossible to you. If something is impossible to you, you have not as much faith as a grain of mustard seed. Crimes, hostility, poverty, wars, and especially so-called incurable illness are all the end result of a lack of faith. . . .
>
> Faith is judgment in infinity. If you do not know the order of the infinite universe, you have no faith. If you have confidence only in man-made contrivances such as laws, power, knowledge, science, money, drugs and medicines, you have faith only in relativity, not in infinity. Since all relative judgment is transitory and of little value, you should learn the structure of the infinite, the eternal creator.
>
> The structure of the infinite is omnipotent, omniscient, and omnipresent. The infinite is almighty and is another name for God. Since God made everything, so disease is a creation of God too. Health is also a creation of God. God manifests in twos everywhere; 'disease and health' is one of such manifestations. Man has the freedom to choose disease rather than health. However, we can choose health at any time. To do this, we have to learn and understand the order of the universe. In other words, we have to be free man instead of sensorial man because sensorial man tends to choose to be sick rather than healthy. This is because sensorial man chooses foods for his pleasure, but free man chooses foods for his spiritual growth. The foods for spiritual growth are of vegetal origin, not animal. Our spirit can develop when we are eating quiet and gentle vegetables, but not if we eat active and red-blooded animals.
>
> Cancer, therefore, is God's creation by which man will learn how to be free from sickness. Until the sick learn this, cancer can never be cured.

Those who were once cured from cancer by the macrobiotic diet and became cancerous again are mostly those who cannot be cured. Thus Ohsawa wrote in *Zen Macrobiotics* (p. 9) twenty years ago:

> No disease is incurable for God, creator of this infinite universe, the kingdom of freedom, happiness, and justice. Nevertheless, there are some sick people who cannot be cured, and who cannot be taught to cure themselves.
>
> Sick people incessantly express the wish for a cure; they claim to have the will to rid themselves of disease at any cost. Will of this variety is merely a desire to escape from the status quo – defeatism. It reveals an unwillingness to accept the eternal order in life, the order that oscillates between difficulty and pleasure, disease and health. To exist in a static state that includes only the one and not the other is impossible. We must continually recreate our own happiness by recognizing and curing disease at every instant of our lives.
>
> Many a man wishes to be cured by others or by some mechanical device, all the while bypassing his own involvement and personal responsibilty, the cause of his disease.

In other words, one who is cured of cancer by the macrobiotic diet but without deep self-reflection that he himself (his ego) is the cause of cancer, that his ego desire grew too far beyond the order for health (which is to live simply, eating mostly grains and vegetables), is not cured.

November 1980

Cooking with Love

I received a letter from an old friend recently. He said, "I have eaten food prepared by many different macrobiotic cooks and only occasionally have I tasted food cooked with love. So many cooks are striving for balance, proper ingredients, etc. If they would only cook with love then there would be no need to worry about all of these things."

He gave the example of his mother's birthday cake which everybody liked and which brought the party a great joy and happiness.

I agreed with his thought, "Love must be the first step." However, I realized his thought might be going too much the other way. In other words, he overlooked the fact that cooking with a striving for balance and proper ingredients is love too.

I know a lady who has a great love. Her love is so great that she thinks about the whole of humanity or heavenly gods when she cooks, and forgets whether she added salt or not, how much miso she put in already, etc., so that her miso soup is sometimes too salty and other times has no taste.

Since she has a great love, she worries often about her friends during cooking. As a result, her mind leaves the kitchen, which sometimes gives her cooking a strange taste.

To me she has too much love, and lacks concentration on immediate things – such as fire on the stove, vegetables and grains in the pots, taste and color of what she is cooking, what is

65

left over from previous meals, what kind of foods others are wanting from my cooking today, etc.

She will be much happier if she starts with smaller love rather than larger love such as heavenly love.

George Ohsawa's 87th Birthday

George Ohsawa was born October 18, 1893. He wrote of his birth in *Kusa,* a magazine he published in India in 1954 before he came to America.

In the ancient capital of Japan, Kyoto, the center of Buddhism founded some 1300 years ago by the Buddhist Emperor Kanmu, there are more than 400 temples and almost all the headquarters of the various sects among them. This capital of Buddhism is surrounded by beautiful green mountains with many temples and pagodas on their slopes and tops.

At the western extremity of the city and at the foot of Mt. Atago there is a big emerald river, serpenting quietly into the Kyoto basin after rolling in zigzag torrents and rapids through rocky valleys covered by dark green woods interspersed with crimson burning azaleas in the spring. On the banks and mountains on both sides of this deep emerald-green serpenting flow at the entrance of the basin, there are thousands and thousands of cherry trees which will blossom in April, reflecting their hue on the surface. There is a long wooden bridge, and on the approach to this there is a very old Buddhist temple.

One day in Autumn 1893, a couple – a young man and his wife – were passing along the moss-grown gates of the temple. They were two adventurers coming from a remote country to try their fortune in the old capital. They were carrying their baggage on their backs and in their hands. Suddenly the young wife asked her husband to pause in front of the gate. She gave birth to a child there.

On October 18, 1980, we – the staff of G.O.M.F. along with friends from Argentina, Japan, and other places – gathered and celebrated Ohsawa's birthday. If he were living he would have been 87 years old. He is in another world now. At this meeting I expressed my thoughts on him briefly; I would like to share them with you, so I wrote them down.

George Ohsawa is known as the founder of the macrobiotic diet in this country as well as Europe and many other countries. However, he was not merely a nutritionist or dietician. He was a thinker, philosopher, salesman, businessman, poet, writer, lecturer, provoker, adventurer, healer, alchemist, prophet, fortuneteller, and, above all, a man of love. He loved all men – the poor as well as the rich, the sick as well as the healthy, the smart as well as the dumb, the suffering as well as the happy.

He said in his monthly magazine published in Japanese: "Man is free, loving, and eternal." He changed the concept of man and he lived it.

From the age of thirty-four (1928) until sixty-three (1957), he published 120 books – four books per year – and many articles in various magazines in France and Japan. His social and economic study of Western countries amounted to 54 volumes. (This is nearly impossible to find now – probably burned by the Japanese military government.) These are not counted in the above number. Furthermore, he wrote letters every day without resting to all his disciples, many scholars, and leaders of the world. He wrote 3600 letters between October 1953 and September 1962 – about 360 letters a year, one letter a day. This is not surprising to you if you are a businessman, but anyone reading them would be surprised because his letters were not just regular postcards, sightseeing cards, but reports on people and places he visited; his experiences curing 'incurable' sicknesses such as tropical ulcers in black Africa; criticisms on social, political, and medical trends; poems; his findings and thoughts on macrobiotic principles and applications, etc. These were sometimes composed of over fifty pages.

Why did he write so much? How could he write so much? His love wouldn't let him sleep. He wrote to unhappy people so that they could be happy. Love for people was his driving energy source. Like his mother, he couldn't pass by emotionless if he saw unhappy or sick people – even if this meant an entire nation.

When Japan began fighting with the world allies, Ohsawa couldn't wait for her complete defeat and misery. He wrote books against the war, hoping to overthrow the government, until he was jailed and sentenced to death by the Japanese police and government. Ohsawa showed no resentment to them but rather he was sorry he couldn't stop the war.

He invited so-called incurable sicknesses to himself such as the tropical ulcers in Africa to prove that macrobiotics could cure and save the unhappy Africans.

His love was not only for humans. He showed love even for bacteria and viruses. He was against killing them in order to relieve pain. This love is the foundation of macrobiotic medicine. He wasted no paper, not even used newspapers or envelopes. He used them again and again. Therefore, he was an original recycler. He scolded us severely if we wasted a grain of rice, any vegetables, salt or oil, etc., because he loved them.

He loved money as well as time, so he wasted no money and no time. If we didn't reply quickly to his letters, he scolded us severely because we were wasting time. In his letters he asked us very difficult questions, keeping us so busy and worried that we had no time or desire for binges. In this way he taught us even in his absence and encouraged us to follow a simple diet.

His love was also sentimental. He loved Japan, the beauty of Japan, beautiful women – and particularly France. He loved intelligence, knowledge, thought, ideas, etc. He loved socially, too. He dreamed of a peaceful one world. He was a federalist – he didn't see any borderlines between nations and races. When I attended his lecture meeting at a university hall in 1940 when Japan, Germany, and Italy signed the treaty against the world allies, he asked the audience, "What is a nation?" His nation was one nation of the universe, where there are no star wars. This was an expression of his social love.

When his love reached ideological love and supreme love it was very severe, piercing, and cold. He gave his whole life to teach us the supreme love. For Ohsawa, life was not worth living without supreme love. If one reaches supreme love, one can live forever. This was the foundation of his macrobiotic teaching. What is supreme love? No exclusivity, he said. Love sickness as you love health. This is his supreme love. Love poverty as you love wealth. Love inconvenience as you love convenience. Love materialism as you love spiritualism. Love the lazy one as you love the hard worker. Love the ugly one as you love the beautiful one. Then there is no divorce. Such was his supreme love. (See "Those Who Love Ugliness" in *Jack and Mitie*, G.O.M.F., 1981, pp. 149-154.)

This is the secret of his medicine.

"We must not kill, not even a microbe. We should consider nothing an enemy. Cancer, allergy, heart disease, mental illness, criminality, juvenile delinquency, war-prone government – all are amusing disciplines that our invisible or absent Director-Instructor, the Infinite, continually confronts us with to unveil and fortify our supreme judgment (love).

"Why do civilized people consider these trials insufferable? Why are they so exclusive?" (*Macrobiotics: The Way of Healing*, formerly *Cancer and the Philosophy of the Far East*, G.O.M.F., 1984.)

His 'exclusivity' is a synonym for dualism which, according to him, is the basic difference between Western and Eastern medicine. Exclusivity is the social expression of the sixth stage of judgment, while dualism is the conscious expression of the sixth stage. "All who see or believe in only one side of the coin (good or evil, body or soul, sentimental or intellectual) are dualistic, exclusive, and quarrelsome. Only those who see that the two sides of phenomena, visible and invisible, are front and back or beginning and end of One Reality can embrace any antagonistic situation, see its complementarity, and help others to do the same – thereby establishing peace and harmony. All who are quarrelsome, all who find anything intolerable in this world are dualistic."

Dualistic thinking and the monistic mentality respond to cancer in entirely different ways, as Ohsawa describes in *Macrobiotics: The Way of Healing*:

> Civilized people consider cancer the most terrible curse to which human society has ever been subjected. Such a fear-crazed attitude is exclusive, lonely, and egocentric. Such fear and hostility become greater and greater and are eventually transformed into aggressive action. Mobilizing all the physical and intellectual means at his disposal (both moral and immoral) in order to destroy his dreaded enemy cancer, man risks no less than his own simultaneous destruction since his cancer and his body are nourished at the same source.
>
> Primitive people who live in accord with the dialectical monistic philosophy are also surprised at the appearance of cancer. But they feel neither fear nor hostility. They are sorry to have caused so much trouble. When scolded with cancer, they examine themselves very deeply in order to discover what they have done to deserve this reprimand.

In short, such dualistic thinking which acknowledges outside elements – viruses, pollution, bacteria, etc. – as the causes of disease has led to the development of symptomatic medicine. Since dualistic thinking belongs to the sixth stage of judgment, which is next to supreme judgment, even distinguished medical doctors stop in this stage. Such an example is Dr. Schweitzer of Africa. He was a great man but he did not reach supreme love. Therefore, he observed symptomatic medicine.

Ohsawa taught us that "love your enemy" is still dualistic. Real love is a state of mind where you find no enemy.

However, Ohsawa's greatness is in the fact that he applied this supreme love in the field of medicine - which is to say monistic, nondualistic medicine, based on totality or oneness which he expressed as the order of the universe. He called this a dialectic medicine.

In *Macrobiotics: The Way of Healing* he states, "As a consequence I am able to declare here once and for all that symptomatic medicine will never cure cancer. Nor will it ever truly cure any disease, not even a common cold."

When I lectured in Europe in May 1980, I said that even macrobiotics cannot cure cancer. One member of the audience asked me after my lecture, "Do you oppose Ohsawa's thought? Ohsawa said there is no incurable disease." I couldn't answer him but I never thought I opposed Ohsawa. Now I understand. If the macrobiotic diet is applied symptomatically, macrobiotic medicine is symptomatic medicine too. Therefore, it cannot cure cancer. This is the meaning of Ohsawa's saying. That is my meaning when I said that even the macrobiotic diet cannot cure cancer.

If one wishes to cure any disease, one must reach the mentality that disease is a sign that we are doing something wrong - violating the order of man in daily life, especially in eating and drinking. Unless we reflect deeply on this fact and reach the awareness that we are always in the infinite totality (by understanding the spiralic concept of the universe - that is to say, monistic thinking) there will be no real cure of any disease, especially cancer. This differentiates macrobiotic medicine from modern medicine, and even from most so-called Oriental medicine.

Ohsawa grew up with the samurai spirit, influenced by his father, relatives, and especially his mother. With the combination of this samurai spirit and his love, he reached the concept of Justice. Justice is one of the most important moods behind his thoughts and actions.

The Seventh Condition
of Health

As I wrote in the last article, Ohsawa was a man of love. Due to this love, he started his teaching of the macrobiotic diet to cure sick people. Due to this love, he demonstrated against the military government of Japan, risking his life to try and prevent World War II. Due to this love, he taught macrobiotic principles and diet throughout the world. Due to this love, he went to black Africa and invited tropical ulcers to himself to prove macrobiotics could cure the disease. Due to this love, he worked on his mission and studied in thousands of books, without personal amusements or family life.

Although Ohsawa was such a great man of love, he often scolded his wife, students, or even audiences severely if they did not understand 'no exclusivity', 'gratitude', etc. His scolding was so severe that many students left him. Some even hated him. Why did this happen? This happened because his love was a manifestation of justice, the justice of infinity. Even in his early book *Life and Environment*, published March 1, 1942 (during the war), he said, "I like nature, I love nature, and I respect the justice of nature – although I often violate the law of nature, knowingly or unknowingly. . . "

In 1941, the year Japan entered World War II, Ohsawa wrote a book called *Standing at the Health Front*. In this book, comparing the health conditions of Americans, Germans, English, and Japanese, Ohsawa was warning the Japanese military government that Japan would be defeated due to its failing health if the Japanese did not change their diet back to their traditional diet. On the back cover of this book Ohsawa predicted that Japanese military leaders would be prosecuted as war criminals.

Ohsawa was not a mere prophet, however. He showed how to improve health from his years of experience teaching macrobiotics and healing sick people. He compiled a definition of health during the time he was working at Shoku Yo Kai (the macrobiotic association founded by the disciples of Sagen Ishizuka). In the appendix of this small booklet, he wrote his six conditions of health:

Physical conditions
1. Never tired, never catch cold. Always ready to work.
2. Good appetite. Happy with simplest foods.
3. Good, deep sleep. Fall asleep within 3 minutes after going to bed and wake up after 4–5 hours. No dreams, no movement during sleep.

Psychological conditions
4. Good memory. Never forgets. Can memorize fifty thousand personal names.
5. Happy from morning to night. Appreciate everything.
6. Live with egoless spirit. There is no selfishness. Devote whole life to truth and the happiness of others.

Four of the above conditions of health have been the same for years. However, he changed the fifth and sixth conditions considerably when he came to America and published *Zen Macrobiotics* in 1960 (later published by The Ohsawa Foundation in 1965).

"Condition 5 – Good Humor. Freedom from anger. A man of good health should be cheerful and pleasant under any circumstance. One should be without fear and suffering. With more difficulties and enemies, such a man will be even more happy and brave and enthusiastic. Your appearance, your voice, your behavior, and even your criticism should distribute deep gratitude and thankfulness to all those who are in your presence."

He changed the next condition more drastically:

"Condition 6 – Smartness in Thinking and Doing. A man who is in good health should have the faculty of correct thinking, judging, and doing with promptness and smartness. Promptness is the expression of freedom. Those who are prompt, speedy, and precise and those who are ready to answer to any challenge or accident or necessity are in good health."

Ohsawa qualified for this condition very well. His action was very fast and smart. Furthermore, his responses and criticisms to all events or opinions were very quick and deep. However, he was not satisfied with this condition. He added one more thing to this sixth condition. That is to say, "A man who is in good health should have the ability to establish order everywhere in daily life. Beauty of action or form is an expression of the order of the infinite universe. Health and happiness are also the expressions of the order of the infinite universe translated in our daily life."

In 1962 he added another condition, written in letters to his students at Nippon Centre Ignoramus in Tokyo (G.O.L. 3641, 3668, 3678, 3695, 3696, 3697, 3698, 3704, and 3803). A digest translation of the above letters follows:

"I left Japan at the age of sixty and visited India, Africa, Europe, America, and even the countries of the Vikings, teaching macrobiotics for ten years. Now I am almost seventy years old which is an age people rarely attain, according to Confucius. As one of my 70th year birthday presents, I received a big gift; that is, the seventh condition of health.

"I compiled six conditions of health thirty years ago, and nobody corrected them. Now I have found the seventh condition. This is the gift I received from heaven for the work I did, risking my life, for the last ten years. This is one of my biggest gifts received from heaven. Due to adding the seventh condition, my previous health valuation was changed completely.

Condition	Points – then	Points – now
1st	10	5
2nd	10	5
3rd	10	5
4th	20	10
5th	20	10
6th	30	10
7th	–	55

"What a slow thinker I am. I needed to be seventy years old in order to find the seventh condition. How pitiful and dumb I am. This finding was inspired by an incident concerning one of my students, G. He was one of my oldest students. He attended my seminars more than twenty times. One day at our meeting, he said, 'My children are lying to you because they are afraid to be scolded by you.' I was so surprised hearing this that I couldn't find any words. What a mentality he has. If his children are lying, he should talk with them. He has no shame for his children's lying. Due to this mentality, he has never been healthy. In other words, he was lacking the seventh condition of health although he has been following macrobiotics for thirty years or more.

"The seventh condition of health is far more important in comparison to the other six conditions. In fact, all other conditions are included within the seventh condition.

"The seventh condition of health: Justice.

"What is justice?

"Do you live with justice?

"According to the Britannica's *Syntopticon*, there is no absolute justice in this world. There is only relative justice such as legal justice and moralistic justice. According to my definition, justice is simply stated: It is another name for the order of the universe. Therefore, one who lives according to the order of the universe acquires absolute justice.

"There are several concepts which cannot be seen, heard, or told. Justice is such a concept. Freedom, happiness, life, peace, eternity, health, harmony, integrity, beauty, and truth are concepts nobody has adequately explained. Everybody wants them, but instead they find and stay with their opposites – unhappiness, death, sickness, quarrels, war, ugliness, lies, anger, hate, etc. People are busy with how to find those things which make them unhappy, unfree, and unjust in the end.

"In this world, there are visible, tangible things and invisible, intangible things. Some people think invisible things do not exist. Democritus, Aristotle, Descartes, Locke, Darwin, etc., belong to this group. They are materialists. There are other people who say that intangible and invisible things are reality. Lao Tsu, Chan Tse, Buddha, Nagarjuna, and Christ belong to this type.

"These two types of thought have been disputed for over two thousand years. At the twentieth century, some of the materialists started to realize that visible things might be produced from the invisible world. However, the majority of people still believe the former concept.

"The macrobiotic concept combines the above two concepts. The world we see and feel is the visible world which is governed by the yin yang antagonism and complementarity. This visible world came from the invisible world. In other words, the visible world (materialistic world) is a part of the invisible world. The governing law of the invisible world is the order of the universe. Another name is justice.

"In our life, realizing justice is the most important condition for being healthy and happy. Lao Tsu said when justice is forgotten, morals, law enforcement, medicine, etc., develop. In other words, if men follow the order of the universe, morals, law enforcement, and medicine are not necessary. Therefore, I put this justice as the seventh condition of health.

"I tried to cure many sick people in my fifty years of macrobiotic teaching. One who is cured easily always understands and tries to observe the justice of nature. One who doesn't understand and refuses to understand is never cured.

"Living is a miracle. Life is the biggest miracle. The fact that we are living is proof that we have the ability to perform a miracle. People are always looking for miraculous power, overlooking the fact that we have such a power. One who understands this fact will cure the sick. One who lives with the 'spirit of miracle' is one who has achieved the seventh condition of heath. The realization of 'miracle' is justice in this visible world. Curing the sick is a small part of that miracle.

"At last, the seventh condition of health is attained by one who has justice in his thinking and doing. Such a person will have the following mentality:

1. He is never angry. Appreciates everything, even the greatest difficulties and unhappiness.
2. He is never afraid.
3. He never says, 'I am tired' or 'I am lost.'
4. He appreciates any foods, even distasteful cooking.
5. He sleeps deeply, without dreams. Four to five hours is enough.
6. He never forgets, especially debts and kindness received.

"The above are the six conditions of health I compiled and have taught for thirty years. Now I have added:

7. He has absolute faith in justice – the order of
the universe. One who attains this seventh
condition of health will have the following
mentality:

He does not lie in order to protect himself.

He is accurate and punctual.

He never meets a man he doesn't like.

He never doubts what others say.

He wants to live to find the eternal, highest
value of life.

He is most happy when he finds the order of
the universe in his daily life and in un-
noticeable small things.

He does not spend his life for earning money
but instead he spends his life only for
what he really wants to do.

He spends his whole life to teach the miracle
of life – the order of the universe."

In the last two articles I have written about Ohsawa and how
some of his teaching came about. As you realize, his teaching
did not come in one day but rather from his untiring pursuit of
health and happiness for all and his striving for highest judgment. As he said, his judgment was growing all the time. This
is because he was always humbly learning, accepting his own
mistakes and the criticism of others.

Now he is gone. It is our turn to learn from his teaching, and
at the same time we climb up to an even higher judgment.

The Enemy Concept

Happy New Year 1981

Mankind has reached the year of 1981 – nineteen years until the twenty-first century. What kind of year will it be in 1981? What should we do in 1981? Let me contemplate for awhile.

The year of 1981 will be one of the most critical years for mankind. The possibility of war between Russia and America is almost as great as in 1961, when J.F. Kennedy sent forces to stop Russian ships which were carrying an atomic warhead. War in the Middle East may be the beginning of World War III.

According to some politicians and the majority of people who support it, nuclear weapons are weapons for peace: protection against our enemies. Thus, the first atomic bomb was dropped on Hiroshima and Nagasaki and killed 350,000 innocent people. Today, the American government produces three atomic warheads a day – each of which is twenty or more times as powerful as the bomb used on Hiroshima and Nagasaki. The whole world possesses a total of about fifty thousand nuclear weapons today, according to what the United Nations reports. These nuclear weapons, being twenty times more powerful than the one dropped on Hiroshima, can instantly kill 8.5 billion people – about double the world's population. This is unbelievable, but this is the scene of 1981. What is the cause of this madness or stupidity? To me, this is the result of school education which teaches the concept of 'enemy'.

Another threat for mankind is cancer. At present, death from heart disease is top in this country; however, it is decreasing. One of the biggest problems facing mankind today is cancer, from which the death rate is increasing. Cancer is steadily killing about half a million people every year in America alone. It is not due to this number, but to its mysterious character and the fact that we don't know the cause, that cancer is the most dreadful curse of mankind today.

Scientists consider cancer the enemy of man. Therefore, they try to destroy it at any cost. Their weapons are surgery, radiation, and chemicals. They declare that those weapons are curing cancer in one out of three cases. In reality, they are merely prolonging life five years more – while causing the sick to suffer even more severe pain. As a consequence, Americans spent a total of $3 billion on medications in 1979. What a waste. What a sad world we live in. What is the cause of this? Again, it is the result of school education which teaches the 'enemy' concept. But cancer is not an enemy. It is a warning sign that our way of living is not in tune with nature.

Nuclear weapons, as well as official cancer treatments, have been created by the concept of 'enemy'. As long as this concept remains, there will be no peace or health. There are no enemies in this world. Without reaching this 'no enemy' concept, neither world peace nor health without cancer can exist.

For us, 1981 should be the year to start such an education. Let us work together toward this.

A Night at Vega

During one of the evening lecture meetings at Vega, our macrobiotic study center, in February, I had a guest student who visited her husband here just for the weekend. Her husband had been at Vega since the beginning of the February session. Since she was a new student to macrobiotics, I asked her whether she had any questions. She told me she had difficulty understanding why summer is yang and winter is yin, because things (plants) grow and expand in summer and contract in winter. "If expansion is yin and contraction is yang, summer must be yin and winter must be yang."

Her view on yin and yang interested me very much because she is very active in winter, skiing and jogging. She is not contracted in winter. However, she sees winter as contracted. She is not seeing herself but her surroundings.

I answered the above question in the following way.

"Summer is hot and winter is cold (in the northern hemisphere). Therefore, summer is yang and winter is yin. Expansion of plants in summer is the result of the attraction of yin such as water, potassium, etc., to heat which is yang. Thus yin, not yang, causes the expansion of plants in summer."

She thinks summer is yin because plants expand in summer. This thinking is the result of confusion of cause (in this case heat), effect (in this case the attraction of yin), and result (plant growth). Plants grow in summer not because of yin but rather yang, which attracted yin elements. Therefore, if there are no yin elements available in an area, plants will not grow – as in the desert. In the case of animals, which are yang, summer (yang) attracts yin – water or yin elements such as potassium – but not enough for animals to grow, and animals usually lose weight in summer.

> Yang summer heat $\triangle$ → attracts yin elements
> (water, K, etc.) → plants grow (yin) $\triangledown$.

She thinks winter is yang because plants contract in winter. Again, this thinking is due to the confusion of cause, effect, and result. Winter coldness (yin) causes the expulsion of yin such as water and potassium from plants, which are necessary for plant growth. Winter coldness is the cause, expelling yin is the effect, and contraction is the result.

> Yin winter cold $\triangledown$ → expels yin elements (water, K,
> etc.) → plants stop growing, or contract (yang) $\triangle$.

A similar cause and effect relationship exists between foods and organs. In the macrobiotic view, the stomach and intestines are considered yin organs. Those organs are activated by yang foods such as miso soup, well-cooked vegetables, etc. This is like the situation in which the hot heat of summer activates plants (yin) to grow.

However, the mechanism of how yang foods activate yin organs is a mystery, because yang foods stimulate the yang nerve (parasympathetic nerve), and then this yang nerve stimulates yin organs. According to the yin yang principle, yin and yang attract each other and stimulate each other, and yin and yin or yang and yang repel each other so that they do not stimulate each other. If the yin yang principle is right, why do yang foods stimulate the yang nerve? The mechanism of this can be explained as follows:

There is a layer of so-called glial cells between the capillaries and the nerve cells. All the yin or yang elements of food pass through these glial cells and reach either the parasympathetic or the sympathetic nerve. Strangely enough, the glial cells act as controlling agents. In other words, some glial cells pass through only yang elements (fig. 1). In this case the glial cells are

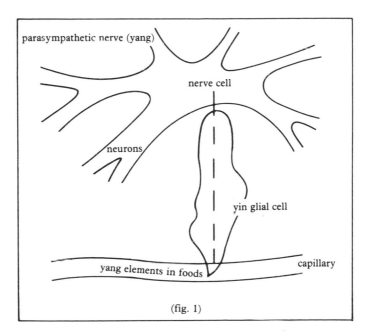

(fig. 1)

yin, so they connect with the yang (parasympathetic) nerve. Yang elements passing through these glial cells stimulate the parasympathetic nerve to produce acetylcholine, which contracts (yang) or activates the stomach, intestine, bladder, etc. (yin organs). However, some glial cells pass through only yin elements (fig. 2). In this case the glial cells are yang, so that these glial cells connect with the yin (sympathetic) nerve. Yin elements passing through the glial cells stimulate the sympathetic nerve to produce norepinephrine, which expands or activates (yin) the heart, liver, kidney, etc. (yang organs).

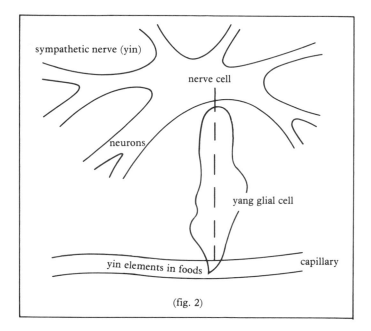

(fig. 2)

This cause and effect can be diagrammed as follows:

Yang foods △ → yin glial cells ▽ → parasympathetic nerve △ → stimulate yin organs ▽ (stomach, intestine, etc.).

Yin foods ▽ → yang glial cells △ → sympathetic
nerve ▽ → stimulate yang organs △ (heart, liver,
kidney, etc.).

Thus, yin acts on yang and vice versa. Always, yin is followed
by yang and yang is followed by yin. This is the order of the
universe.

A simple yin yang question ended up with the above

explanation of a complicated physiological mechanism. The students paused for awhile. Then a student asked an entirely different question:

S_1 – Do you believe in reincarnation?

H – No, I don't believe because I know it.

S_2 – I believe in reincarnation.

H – I don't believe because I know.

S_2 – How do you know?

H – What is your origin? Where do you come from?

The students couldn't answer.

Your origin is what you eat. And the origin of what you eat is light, air, water, minerals . . . the atomic world. The origin of the atomic world is the world of pre-atoms such as electrons, protons, and neutrons. The origin of the pre-atomic world is vibration or energy. The origin of energy is the world of polarization – yin yang. The origin of yin yang is infinity. Our life started from infinity and goes back to infinity after we die. Then we start another life. This is my explanation of reincarnation. Therefore, I know I will come back again to this world because we live in the infinite world.

S_2 – I understand now our physical origin. However, how did we start our individual soul which makes up our character, traits, behavior, etc.?

H – You are asking a question which many thinkers of the East as well as the West have tried in vain to solve since the beginning of civilization. Kukai, a Japanese Buddhist, the founder of the Shingon sect, described our soul in nine stages but did not succeed in solving this question.

Jean-Paul Sartre of France tried to solve it in *Being and Nothingness*. However, I don't think he succeeded. William James and Alfred Adler of America tried to explain the nature of the human soul. However, they have not succeeded in explaining the origin of individual souls.

In my opinion, the reason they failed in solving this problem is that they do not unite body and soul. Unifying body and soul, the macrobiotic concept explains this question very well. The following is my explanation of the individual soul.

First we again go back to the origin of our body. The body is formed by trillions of cells which are transformed from blood cells (1). Blood cells are the products of foods we eat. (Most scientists, except a few, do not agree with this view. However, it is a clear fact that if we don't eat, we have neither blood nor bone marrow.) The foods we eat are vegetal, or products of the vegetal world. Therefore, the first origin of our body is the vegetal world (2). The origin of the vegetal world is the atomic world (3). The origin of the atomic world is the pre-atomic world (4). The origin of the pre-atomic world is energy, such as electromagnetism, gravitation, kinetic energy, potential energy, heat energy, etc. (5). The origin of energy is polarization or yin and yang (6). The origin of polarization is 'the one', infinity, or the 'nothingness' of Lao Tsu (*taikyoku,* or the 'Great Pole' of Chinese philosophy) (7).

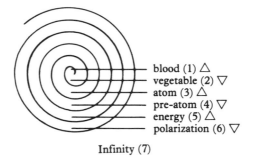

Infinity (7)

This infinity is the ultimate origin of our body. However, the same infinity is also the ultimate origin of our soul. Infinity is I. Infinity or oneness is the primal state of matter and mind. From this oneness or infinity, the material world and the spiritual world branch out. The material and the spiritual world each have seven stages, and the seventh stage is the same one for both: Infinity, universal consciousness, nothingness, or God.

This infinity is like a TV broadcasting company. It sends out all kinds of judgments, thoughts, knowledge, emotions, feelings, etc. The individual soul is like a TV set which, due to individual constitution and condition, tunes in to some of those judgments, thoughts, knowledge, emotions, and feelings. In this way, individual souls build their character, traits, and behavior. Therefore, the origin of the individual soul is infinity. To what judgment, emotion, or feeling we will tune depends on our TV set. And what determines the quality of this TV set is the thoughts, deeds, and diet of our ancestors, parents, and ourselves. Of course, our diet is the most effective factor for the reception of the TV signals.

When we tune to physical judgment, we (as a fetus) have basic instinct. As soon as blood changes to cells, these first cells tune in and receive physical judgment coming from infinity. Then the brain, nervous system, digestive organs, and heart are formed and begin functioning according to the yin yang principle.

When we tune to sensorial judgment, we can distinguish different colors, voices, noises, tastes.

When we tune to sentimental judgment, we can distinguish different emotions such as joy, sadness, hate, resentment, anger, happiness, regret, etc.

When we tune to intellectual judgment, we can study various concepts and knowledge – science, etc.

When we tune to social or economic judgment, we become a socialist, capitalist, communist, politician, etc.

When we tune to philosophical, religious, or dualistic judgment, we divide things into mind and matter, good or bad, right or wrong, friend or enemy, etc.

When we tune to the seventh level of judgment, the voice of infinity and justice, our soul becomes the universal soul and our body becomes infinity. This time, body and soul unite. We can embrace everything.

Our thoughts are not our creation but the creation of infinity. We only pick up a few of them. When we do, we think "We thought." However, all thoughts, all feelings, and all emotions are not ours, but infinity – produced and broadcast. Our brain tunes in to some of them. Then we feel something.

This is my explanation of individual soul. Let me hear your criticism. Our students at Vega were very happy to hear this explanation. One said this was the most wonderful explanation of soul he had ever heard.

Macrobiotic Jackpot

When I arrived at the Sheraton Palace Hotel in San Francisco on March 10th to hear Dr. Anthony Sattilaro and Michio Kushi speak, I saw a short man passing by my side. Realizing this was Dr. Sattilaro, I started to introduce myself. To my surprise, before I could say my name he shook my hand and said, "Hello, Herman." He acted as if we had known each other for a long time. He was very friendly.

He started his speech with gratitude to the teachers of macrobiotics, even me. I was surprised by his honoring me as his teacher because I never taught him. He explained the cancer prevention diet not only from a Western medical point of view but also from the macrobiotic way. To my surprise, he went into quite a bit of detail on Chinese medicine to explain various cancer sicknesses. He ended his speech with a 100 percent recommendation of the macrobiotic diet for cancer. I thought I was dreaming. It is a miracle that he cured his cancer with the macrobiotic diet. However, his faith and recommendation of the macrobiotic diet – as a doctor of Western medicine – is more than a miracle.

Twenty years ago, when Mr. Ohsawa started the macrobiotic lectures in New York City, a young M.D. began the diet. To his surprise, his wife cured her alcoholism by observing macrobiotics too. He then began to recommend macrobiotics to his patients. I had the first American macrobiotic store, in

Greenwich Village, at that time. I had at least ten customers from this doctor every day. A medical doctor's influence is very strong. However, he quit his macrobiotic teaching due to fear of condemnation by the AMA and the loss of his patients. Patients who once learned the diet usually didn't go back to the doctor because they cured sicknesses by themselves, or because they disliked a doctor who didn't give medications. Anyway, he stopped teaching macrobiotics, and probably he quit the diet too. His wife became alcoholic again and they separated soon after. Since then, the macrobiotic movement in this country has never been accepted by medical doctors. Rather, they claimed macrobiotics was the most dangerous diet.

Ohsawa convinced and converted many medical professionals to macrobiotics in Japan. Many of them are helping macrobiotics in Japan today. However, he didn't succeed in countries other than Japan. He tried to convince Dr. Schweitzer by contracting a case of tropical ulcers and curing it macrobiotically. Even by such life-sacrificing effort, no influential medical doctor joined the macrobiotic movement.

Now we have Dr. Sattilaro, an influential medical doctor and the chief executive officer of a big-city hospital, on our side. This is a jackpot, a million dollar jackpot for the macrobiotic movement. He will introduce hundreds of medical professionals to macrobiotics who will in turn convince millions of people of its value. Sean McLean and Bill Bochbracher, the two hitchhikers who introduced Dr. Sattilaro to the diet, must be honored as the most valuable macrobiotic students. Denny Waxman should be honored in the Macrobiotic Hall of Fame next to Michio Kushi.

Even if a hundred cancer cases were cured with the macrobiotic approach, the American medical authorities would not give credit to the diet. However, Dr. Sattilaro's case is different. He is a reputable medical doctor who cured his own 'incurable' cancer by including the macrobiotic diet, under the eyes of many medical professionals. This fact is undeniable. Many medical doctors will apply the macrobiotic diet to their patients. This will bring about a tremendous revolution of medicine. Dr. Sattilaro will stand at the top of that.

I have been wondering how Dr. Sattilaro was able to cure his incurable cancer in such a short time. Even by macrobiotic standards his cure is miraculous and unbelievable. When I heard his lecture, I understood the reason. He is an extremely friendly, open person. He has no exclusivity. Therefore, he picked up the two hippies. With this character, he dared to listen to a layman's words on cancer cure. He started the macrobiotic diet not simply because he was desperate, but because he had no prejudice toward any new idea. If he were closed-minded, he would never have tried macrobiotics; he is an M.D., and macrobiotics has had a very poor reputation in the profession.

His open-mindedness, however, was not the reason. Didn't he worry about criticism which might be given in medical circles? Wasn't he afraid of the condemnation of the AMA because his attitude was so controversial within all the teachings of modern medicine? He may have been. However, in my opinion, he had to stand up and tell the public that he recommends the macrobiotic diet for cancer treatment because he has not only gratitude but also justice.

Dr. Sattilaro could cure his terminal cancer in one year because he had the mind of justice, which is the highest condition of health. In other words, Dr. Sattilaro was never a sick man. His only sickness was physical, caused by poor eating due to his education. Therefore, as soon as he realized his mistake, he could correct the physical condition very easily. He did not need correction in his thinking. His judgment was very high.

This is the reason Dr. Sattilaro cured his cancer, and this is the reason he now teaches macrobiotics to the world. He is a man of justice. That we have such a man at this time is more of a miracle than curing cancer.

May 1981

A Happy Cancer Patient

At the beginning of January 1981, Vega welcomed a cancer patient, a woman from the California high country. She had breast cancer; the left breast was removed last summer and now the right one had started malignancy. She came to see me last October for a consultation on diet. She went home and continued the macrobiotic diet as she understood it. In order to study macrobiotic principles and cooking, she came to Vega.

When she first came she had back pain all night long. If you have ever had such an experience, you know what this means. She couldn't lie on her back on the floor for the pain. Every morning we did Sotai exercises, self-exercise as well as the two-person treatments. A week later, her back pains disappeared. She could sleep all night without pain. What a joy.

One morning she found herself lying on the floor. She could lie on the floor without pain. She was enjoying the diet. She was better every day.

I never heard her complain. She was healthier than most so-called healthy persons. She was a surprise to me. However, the biggest surprise came at the last lecture of that Vega session. I was talking about 'being happy'. I said, George Ohsawa once told us the definition of a happy man. He said a happy man is one who wants to repeat his life from beginning to now, exactly.

As soon as I said this, she said, "Me too!" In fact, she had already confessed her feeling to the other students before my talk that night. Therefore, her thought was not the result of what I said.

I never met a person who was willing to repeat his or her life again exactly the same way. Most people give some conditions they want to change. But she must really be happy.

She is a rare, happy cancer patient.

From Heart Disease to Cancer

I

Heart and cardiovascular diseases have been the number one killer in this country. However, according to U.S. government statistics, the death rate from heart disease decreased 10 percent and the death rate from cardiovascular disease decreased 16 percent in the period from 1960 to 1977.

Does this mean the American health condition is improving?

The American diet has changed very much in the past twenty years. The following five points will describe some of these changes:

1. After Rachel Carson wrote *Silent Spring* in 1962, environmental pollution became a big issue; also, people have become more concerned about food additives, and, generally, people began selecting more unprocessed natural foods free from preservatives or colorings.

2. Ancel Keys conducted a human experiment with 12,000 persons during the period from 1948 to 1960, concluding that heart and cardiovascular diseases are caused by high cholesterol foods. Keys's report was a cover story for *Time* magazine around 1960; at that time Mr. Ohsawa was staying at my apartment in New York City and he liked the report very

much. This report encouraged less consumption in the American diet of high-fat foods such as beef, pork, chicken, eggs, and cheese. It also encouraged the substitution of vegetable oil for fat, unsaturated oil for saturated, margarine for butter, and low fat skim milk instead of regular milk.

3.   The next big change in the American diet was brought by the English doctor Denis Burkitt. He had been working at a hospital in South Africa in the 1950s, and during that time he noticed that a certain tribe had no heart disease for a period of five years. He wondered and searched for the reason. He concluded the natives not only ate less fat (10 percent of total food consumption) but also realized they took a lot of fiber in their diet. He also found that members of the same tribe who adopted the white people's diet (sugar, foods with no fiber, etc.) did suffer from heart and cardiovascular disease. Members of the tribe who ate only traditional foods had no heart or cardiovascular disease.

4.   The effects of cholesterol and fiber have been studied by many scientists. As a result, they concluded the high cholesterol, low fiber diet is one of the most important causes of heart and cardiovascular disease. This new scientific finding led to the publication of *Dietary Goals for the U.S.*, by the Senate Select Committee on Nutrition and Human Needs headed by Senator George McGovern (January 1977). This recommendation was later modified by the FDA due to pressure from the meat, dairy, and sugar industries.

5.   At present the most popular diet for heart diseases is the Pritikin Diet. This program uses no salt or sugar, low amounts of protein and fat (10 percent animal foods), and no oil, except that already present (8 to 10 percent) in prescribed foods – whole grains, vegetables, and fruit. To me, this diet seems very similar to the macrobiotic diet, and very good for most people. However, due to the lack of the yin and yang principle, salt is

prohibited for everyone, and fruit is recommended for everyone. This will be too much yin for certain people and may cause a bad effect.

These dietary changes are the main reason America reduced her death rate from heart disease during the period from 1960 to 1977. However, the American health condition is not improving. The death rate from cancer increased 16 percent during the same period. In other words, death caused by cancer replaced the deaths caused by heart and cardiovascular disease. The government recommended a diet that was for heart disease but not for cancer. The American government should now compile a Dietary Goals for cancer prevention and cure.

Why did heart and cardiovascular disease decrease while cancer increased? Heart disease decreased due to the reduced consumption of fats and the increased consumption of fiber. Cancer increased due to the increasing consumption of sugar and chemicals. However, in my opinion, the biggest cause is the cutting out of salt.

Nutritionists and the medical profession are afraid of salt. They all oppose the use of salt. One reason the elimination of salt is advised is that most people consume many animal foods and processed foods, all of which contain large amounts of salt or sodium. Therefore, they do not need salt either in cooking or as a condiment on the table. However, salt is the strongest alkaline forming food; without it, we lose much of our immunity, our control against cancer cell growth. (Salt is yang – it opposes malignant cell growth which is yin.) Vegetarians and those who eat no processed foods do not get enough sodium to maintain an alkaline condition of the body fluids, or the proper balance between K/Na (potassium/sodium) of the inter- and intracellular fluids, if they don't use salt in cooking.

Without salt, cancer will never be controlled. However, refined salt is not good. Salt should be used mainly in cooked food, so that sodium is combined with carbohydrates, proteins, or fats in order to keep it from inhibiting heart action. Contrary to salt in cooking, raw table salt changes the sodium content of the blood too fast. This inhibits heart movement and is one cause of heart trouble.

When people change their diet, they change their cooking too. They buy grains, fresh vegetables, and fruit. If they do not use any salt in cooking, there will be almost no sodium in the diet. This will upset the balance of sodium and potassium in the body fluids. Also when people change their diet, they stop eating snack foods such as pretzels, nuts, or potato chips. This further reduces sodium intake. In other words, Americans reduced their salt consumption in order to prevent heart disease, but this was done without consideration of the food selection.

When eating animal foods or foods that have been processed, added salt is not necessary; when foods are fresh and no animal products are consumed, adding salt in cooking is necessary.

Changes in Na and K Content of Peas

Food (100 gram edible portion)	Na (mg)	K (mg)
Fresh peas	0.9	380
Frozen peas	100.0	160
Canned peas	230.0	180

Source: U.S. Dietary Goals, Senate Select Committee on Nutrition, 1977.

In the macrobiotic diet, miso and soy sauce are used for condiments instead of salt. These two contain a lot of sodium but also potassium and protein, thereby supplying not only salt but also essential amino acids (especially vitamin B_{12}) which become more important when animal foods are eliminated. Furthermore, miso and soy sauce are strong alkaline forming foods. Therefore, they would be better to use than salt.

Modern medicine knows the cause of heart disease but is still looking for the cause of cancer, although statistics suggest that diet may be the main cause. According to the 1980 Handbook of the American Cancer Society, 58.04 percent of all deaths will be from diet-related diseases including heart disease, stroke, diabetes, cirrhosis of the liver, nephritis and arteriosclerosis combined, and cancer of the breast and colon. Although they admit breast and colon cancer are caused by the high consumption of fats, they still do not consider that diet is the cause of other cancers.

For example, the number one killer is lung cancer. According to cancer authorities, smoking is the cause of lung cancer. In the United States, 100,000 now die in a year as a result of lung cancer and of these about 80,000 (80 percent) are cigarette smokers. Therefore the American Cancer Society claims cigarette smoking causes lung cancer. However, 80 percent of Japanese males smoke, yet their death rate due to lung cancer is second to the lowest in the world. If smoking is the cause of lung cancer, Japanese males should have a high rate of death by lung cancer.

In my opinion, foods and carcinogens in the diet are *initiators* of the lung cancer and smoking is the *promoter*. (The initiator is a substance or force which changes genes in the cells. The promoter makes the malignant cells grow.) Therefore, if the diet is right, lung cancer will never start.

Without knowing the cause of cancer, authorized medicine has three treatments for cancer. All of them are designed to try and destroy or eliminate cancer cells: surgery, radiation, and chemotherapy. According to official reports, these treatments approved by the AMA cure one out of three cancer cases. This 'cure' means that patients live for five years after the cancer cells are eliminated. In other words, the patients do not necessarily become healthy (or even less, happy), but the treatment just eliminates the cancer cells. Usually the cancer appears again, sooner or later. Not only are these treatments effective in only one-third of cancer cases, they also produce bad side effects. Many people do not like these treatments. They would rather receive unorthodox treatment, such as offered by many of the clinics that are located outside the U.S.

II

In my opinion, all cancer treatments – official, unofficial, Hoxsey's, Gerson's, Krebiozen, Interferon, Laetrile, and Thymosin – are all symptomatic treatments. Even if they succeed, they are not a true cure because they are not curing the basic cause of cancer. In fact, science does not yet know the cause of cancer.

What is the cause of cancer? What is the factor changing DNA and RNA? The American Cancer Society predicted that 58.04 percent of all deaths in 1980 would be related to diet. According to them, breast and colon cancer are related to diet. The ACS does not count diet as the cause of lung cancer; instead they claim smoking as the cause. As mentioned before, this is not true in the case of the Japanese. Their death rate is high in stomach cancer. Why don't Japanese males die from lung cancer?

In the United States, 100,000 people now die annually as a result of lung cancer and 80 percent of these are cigarette smokers. Naturally, the ACS claims cigarette smoking causes lung cancer. Then what is the cause for the 20 percent of non-smokers who have lung cancer, as well as for the Japanese males?

The cause of cancer was demonstrated by Japanese immigrants to the United States. I am one of them. The Japanese have second to the highest rate of death caused by stomach cancer, but a low incidence of cancer of the breast and colon. On the other side of the Pacific, in the United States, there is a high incidence of breast and colon cancer and a lower incidence of stomach cancer.

The Japanese who moved to Hawaii began to eat chicken, beef, cheese, etc., rather than fish, which has less fat. They also consume sugar in the form of refreshments or soft drinks instead of in sweet bean cakes or vegetable or fish cooking. The longer they stay in the United States, the more they consume American-type foods. When they eat American-type foods, they have a higher incidence of colon and breast cancer, which are the cancers most common in America.

Dr. Gio Gori, Deputy Director of the National Cancer Institute, informed the Senate Select Committee in July of 1976:

> There is a strong correlation between dietary fat intake and incidence of breast and colon cancer. As the dietary intake of fat increases, you have an almost linear increase in the incidence of breast and colon cancer. Colon cancer has also been shown to correlate highly with the consumption of meat, even though it is not clear whether the meat itself or its fat content is the real correlating factor. Seventh Day Adventists and Mormons have a restricted fat and meat intake when compared to other populations living in the district and, as indicated, they suffer considerably less from some forms of cancer, notably breast and colon.

According to Japanese doctors K. Chishima and K. Morishita, body cells (soma cells) are transformed from blood cells (red globules). Therefore the cause of cancer is malignant transformation from blood to cells. According to Ohsawa and Ohmori, Japanese macrobiotic leaders, the cause of cancer is excess consumption of sugar and animal foods such as cheese, fish, meat, and eggs. They believe those foods make cancer cells from blood. However, they did not explain the mechanism of this transmutation.

III

In *The Greatest Battle* (Random House, 1976, p. 41), Dr. Ronald J. Glasser explains well how cancer cells develop:

> We know today, and it makes absolute biological sense, that it is the nucleoproteins, with their bases seemingly so safely for billions of years locked away inside the nucleus of cells, that carcinogens injure. It has been proved through a decade of precise, laboriously controlled research that no matter what the carcinogens, chemical or physical, no matter how diverse they may seem to be on the surface – benzopyrene or aniline dyes, asbestos or x-ray – they all share that one same basic property. They all affect the cell's genetic material by getting into the cell and, once inside, working their way into the nucleus, where they either bind to or simply destroy sections of parts of the cell's nucleic acids. We know that in large doses, carcinogens kill cells. They are all basically intracellular poisons. In smaller doses, because of their unique affinity for genetic material, they do not kill cells, they cause them to mutate, and it is this mutagenic nature of carcinogens that causes cancer.

According to Dr. Glasser, the carcinogens which normal cells are exposed to are called the initiators, and the irritants causing the malignant transformation the promoters. His conclusion on initiators and promoters is very important (p. 38): "This meant that once a cell is exposed to a low but critical level of a carcinogen, it becomes premalignant and stays that way, never reverting back to normal, always ready on exposure to some irritant – no matter how long into the future, no matter how distant in time from its original contact with the premalignant levels of carcinogen – to turn overtly malignant." It seems to me that Dr. Glasser's thought on cancer is right. However, he does not explain very well what the initiators and promoters are.

In my opinion, the initiators are carcinogens (chemicals, radiation, asbestos, etc.) and promoters are smoking; strong acid forming foods such as sugar; and fatty foods such as meat, fish, eggs, and cheese, resulting in an acidic condition of the internal fluids. According to modern physiology, body fluids (consisting of inter- and intracellular fluids) must be slightly alkaline. If they turn to acid, cells will die. If brain cell fluids reach a pH of 6.9, we have coma. If we maintain a slightly acidic condition but not acidic enough to kill cells, then this acidic fluid will promote the growth of malignant cells, or produce malignant cells. In other words, acidic intracellular fluid will be the promoter in cancer formation and growth.

What, then, is the cause of the acidic condition of body fluids? All foods can be divided into two groups, namely, acid forming and alkaline forming foods. Excessive eating of acid forming foods will cause an acidic condition in the body fluids.

Among these foods, beans and grains are only slightly acid forming; whole grains especially are very slightly acid forming. Animal foods and sugar are the strongest acid forming foods among those listed on page 106. Therefore, abstinence from those foods is the best recommendation for preventing and stopping the development of cancer.

According to Oriental philosophy, everything can be divided into two characteristics – yin and yang. Yin is expansive (upward movement, cold, light weight, towards the violet or cool end of the spectrum, etc.), while yang is contractive (downward movement, heat, heavy, red or warm side of the spectrum, etc). Acid forming foods dominated by yin such as fats, oils, and sugar cause cancers in the higher parts of the body, because yin goes in an upward direction. On the

Acid Forming Foods

in approximate order of yin to yang
both vertically and within each category

Most chemicals, medicinal drugs, psychedelic drugs, sugar, candy, soft drinks, vinegar, saccharin, vodka, some wine, whiskey, sake, beer

Corn oil, olive oil, sesame oil, peanut butter, sesame butter

Cashews, peanuts, almonds, chestnuts

Soybeans, green peas, tofu, white beans, pinto beans, kidney beans, black beans, chickpeas, red beans (azuki)

Macaroni, spaghetti

Corn, oats, barley, rye, wheat, rice, buckwheat

Shellfish, eel, carp, white meat fish, cheese, fowl, red meat, tuna, salmon, eggs

contrary, acid forming foods dominated by yang such as animal products will produce cancers in the lower areas of the body, because yang goes downward. Foods between them such as beans and grains (and white rice, white flour products, shellfish, etc.) promote cancer at the center of the body.

Although beans and grains are acid forming foods, they are indispensable to our diet in order to maintain health. They are sources of carbohydrates, proteins, fats, minerals, vitamins, and enzymes. In China and Japan these have been considered principal foods for thousands of years. However, being acid forming, grains and beans need alkaline forming foods in order to maintain balanced health.

In order to alkalize the blood and body fluids, one must eat

Alkaline Forming Foods

in approximate order of yin to yang
both vertically and within each category

Natural wine, natural sake, cola, cocoa, fruit juices, coffee, tea (dyed), mineral water, soda water, well water

Honey, mustard, ginger, pepper, curry, cinnamon

Tropical fruits, dates, figs, lemons, grapes, raisins, bananas, peaches, currants, pears, plums, oranges, watermelon, apples, cherries, strawberries

Potatoes, eggplant, tomatoes, shiitake, taro potatoes, cucumber, sweet potatoes, mushrooms, spinach, asparagus, summer squash, broccoli, celery, cabbage, pumpkin, onions, turnips, daikon, nori, hijiki, carrots

Squash seeds, pumpkin seeds, sunflower seeds, sesame seeds

Wakame, kombu, millet, lotus root, burdock, dandelion root, jinenjo

Bancha tea, kuzu tea, grain beverage, dandelion tea, mu tea, ginseng tea

Sesame salt, soy sauce, miso, umeboshi, salt

alkaline forming foods. However, there are yin and yang alkaline forming foods. Therefore it is important to select yin alkaline forming foods for overly yang persons or for more yang cancers (such as colon cancer). A reddish face is usually the result of an overly yang diet with too much animal foods and sodium (although sometimes this is caused by too much alcohol); therefore, such a person will be balanced with yin vegetables. A pale, anemic person (or a yin cancer) needs yang alkaline forming foods such as carrots, burdock, lotus root, miso, ginseng tea, mu tea, etc.

Fruits are excellent alkaline forming foods; however, an excess of fruit sugar (fructose) turns to fat, causing arterial blockage. Therefore, fruits should not be overeaten. Honey and maple syrup are alkaline forming. However, they are rich in disaccharides just like refined sugar. They are very yin and will upset sugar metabolism. Therefore they should not be overconsumed, especially in the case of cancer patients. Coffee is alkaline forming but very yin. Yin cancer patients should avoid it. These yin foods may encourage the expansive spreading (metastasis) of cancers.

IV

The April 1981 issue of *Science* had an article entitled "Why Do Cancer Cells Run Amok?" by Ben Patrusky. In this article are the questions most asked by modern civilized people; every cancer scientist is looking for the answer in order to save millions of cancer victims or to win fame as the most distinguished man of today. In my opinion, the question is simple but can't be answered by scientists because they are looking for the answer without acknowledging the simple fact that all cells, whether normal or malignant, have to eat foods. The secret of cancer is in these foods.

With this belief, I will try to answer the questions posed by this writer, hoping my thoughts may inspire some scientists to investigate the foods consumed by cells.

Why do cells not grow indefinitely?

Our body cells consist of proteins, amino acids, sugars, fats, minerals, water, enzymes, vitamins, etc. Some of them work expansively (yin) and some work contractively (yang). If expansive elements dominate over contractive, the cells grow larger. If contractive elements dominate, cells grow smaller. Note: whether cells grow larger or smaller depends on the proportion between the amount of expansive elements (such as K, P, S, Cl, O, and N) and contractive elements (such as Na, Mg, and H).

However, this growth is not indefinite, because growth relies on the supply of food to the cells. The food for the cells comes by osmosis through the surface membranes of the cells. In order to supply enough food, therefore, the surface area of the membrane must be large enough for foods to pass through and to adequately sustain the activity of each cell. If r is the radius of a cell, assuming the cell is spherical, and A is the surface area of a cell and V is the volume of a cell, then between r, A, and V there are the following relationships:

$$V = \frac{4}{3} \pi r^3 \qquad A = 4 \pi r^2$$

This shows that the radius of a cell is related to its volume by the power of three, and to its surface area by the power of two. In other words, the volume grows at a faster rate than the surface area as the radius increases. When cells reach a certain size (the point of equilibrium), foods passing through the surface are not enough to support the volume of the cell and it stops growing. This is the automatic control of normal cell growth.

Why do cells divide?

When the surface area and volume of cells reach equilibrium, the cells stop growing. However, if expansive elements dominate over contractive elements in the food that cells are consuming after growth stops, the expansive or centrifugal power divides the cells. This is cell division. When cells divide, the surface area is much larger in relation to the volume, so cells grow. When cells reach the point of equilibrium and expansive elements continue to dominate, cells divide again.

Why can malignant cells grow indiscriminately?

Malignant cells also need foods to live and grow. However, their foods are different from those required by normal cells. Malignant cells can sustain their life on the waste products of normal cells. Furthermore, malignant cells need no oxygen. This is the reason cancer cells are almost impossible to kill (see "The Cells That Would Not Die," April 1981 issue of *Science*). The size of malignant cells is also restricted by the ratio of surface area A to volume V. However, malignant cells receive more acidic nutrients, which are expansive, and so malignant cells grow and divide much faster than normal cells.

What causes normal cells to change to malignant?

I agree with Dr. Glasser's opinion that carcinogens are the initiators of cancer. However, cancer does not start right away after initiation by carcinogens. There has to be a promoter which develops cancer cells already initiated by carcinogens. These two concepts of cancer formation, initiator and promoter, explain cancer mechanism very well.

In my opinion, the acidic condition of intracellular fluid is the strongest promoter. The cause of this acidic condition is poor breathing and the consumption of too many acid forming as compared to alkaline forming foods.

October 1981

Summer Lecture Trip 1981

Macrobiotic Families

It is the most pleasurable and rewarding part of the tour to meet old friends, especially when their families are healthier and happier. Our first stop in Salt Lake City gave us such a joy. However, this is not often the case. There always exist some difficulties between husband and wife. Mrs. A. is too yang. Therefore, she likes to cook with less salt. This makes her husband and child too yin. He lost his sex appetite, and the child was cranky. Since he had no sex appetite, he was always working overtime without spending much time with his wife. If this continues too long, the marriage will meet crisis.

On this trip I visited many macrobiotic centers where people were afraid of salt. They have not learned enough about cooking. Cooking must make food taste sweet with the use of salt, soy sauce, or miso. Without these condiments, the taste is bland and the food gives less energy. At the beginning of the macrobiotic teaching, people used too much salt. Now we have the reaction to it. We should not observe the diet only by reaction but also with good judgment.

An old student of mine who was divorced from his wife a couple of years ago invited us to come and give lectures and cooking classes. I was so happy to see he had a beautiful and gentle new wife, living in a nice house. He said he will not make the same mistake again. What is the mistake he made? I think it

111

was a too idealistic expectation from his former wife. However, he is making the same mistake again. He is too demanding, expecting too much from his wife. According to her, he always tells her that she has eaten too much dairy foods in the past. Hearing such words once or twice will be okay; however, hearing it all the time will be torture to the newlywed wife. She cannot change her past eating habits. Such an attitude helps nothing but to break up the marriage relationship. This attitude in men is the result of a too idealistic character; men tend to be idealistic, which leads to a fanatic attitude. Since macrobiotics is a very idealistic way of viewing life, many macrobiotic men therefore have a tendency to a fanatic attitude. Fanatic attitudes always bring us some difficulties. Mr. B. is also an idealistic, fanatical man, so he had big trouble with his previous wife. He has another girlfriend. However, he will have trouble with this girl because he is too fanatic, too extreme, and he lacks generosity.

At the Mid-Atlantic Summer Camp, I met a couple who thanked me and said my teaching had made their marriage happy. She said that one night when she was very much confused about her relationship with her husband, she dreamed of my teaching and solved her problem. This was my unexpected joy on this tour. I experienced a similar joy at Spokane, Washington. One couple who had three children came to see me that night for a consultation. They said they attended the French Meadows Summer Camp in 1977 before they were married. She said I told her, "You better marry him." She not only did so, but also made three children.

Although they are a very happy couple, they had a problem. She is too attached to the children, which makes her husband jealous. Cornellia advised her that they should go out together once a week, giving the children to a babysitter. They are happy again after the talk.

Macrobiotic Farmers in the U.S.A.

Finally I found some macrobiotic farmers. They don't use any chemicals in their garden. They don't even use a big tractor. The farmers are Mr. and Mrs. Tom McDonald, who are living in Trumansburg, New York, population of about a thousand, located near Ithaca. They bought thirty acres of farmland here six years ago and have been farming successfully since then. As soon as we rested enough at their home, Shelley took us to their farm five miles out of town where they are producing all kinds of vegetables – kale, cucumbers, cabbage, squash, scallions, onions, carrots, and one grain: rye. Their main produce is cucumbers and cabbage which are the material for their famous Samurai Pickles. It is so cold in winter that of course they cannot farm. Therefore, pickling in winter is a very good idea. Tom had just finished planting autumn cucumbers when we arrived, she said. She will be very busy this autumn and winter, harvesting and pickling those cucumbers.

The next day it was cloudy and cold. Over forty people came for Cornellia's cooking class and my lecture. This is amazing that such a small town can draw so many people to the macrobiotic events. This is due to the influence of Tom, Shelley, and her sister Kay. They have three children and are a happy family. I hope their happiness continues.

American East and West

It was so humid when we arrived at Lane's home in New Jersey from Washington, D.C. I was curious about why the East is humid and the West (except a few places in Oregon and Washington) is dry.

I reasoned as follows: The East is humid because there are more trees and grasses growing, while the West is more of a desert. Why this difference? Plants grow more in the East because the soil is finer, due to the fact that it is older than western soil – having passed ice ages and rains. Contrary to the East, the West is newer land and therefore there are more rocks. There are all kinds of rock formations in the West: the Black Hills and Badlands of South Dakota; the Bighorn National Forest and Shell Canyon of Wyoming; Zion National Forest of Utah; and the Grand Canyon of Arizona are a few of them.

The difference in natural environment produces the difference in human activities and lifestyles. The East started with farming, then industry and commerce. The West started with husbandry and then mining, and stayed that way until many more people moved there to develop agriculture.

In the East, people are formal and conservative. At a macrobiotic summer camp there, people wear white shirts, ties, and dress shoes. In the West, no one wears white shirts and ties at the summer camps. In the East, people are so conservative that macrobiotics is too radical for them. On the contrary, people in the West are so radical that even macrobiotics is too conservative for them.

Driving the car from the West to the East and back, I saw and felt the differences between the two: green and rocks, industry and mining, commerce and agriculture, conservatives and radicals, yin and yang.

The Small is Strong
The Medfly Syndrome

At the beginning of July, a family moved into our Vega Study House from the San Jose area because California Governor Jerry Brown, who had hoped to fight a medfly infestation with ground spraying, agreed reluctantly to permit aerial spraying of the insecticide malathion on July 10th.

Knowing me for a long time and being that her newborn baby was just a week old, this young mother asked me if she and her three children could stay at Vega during this time in order to avoid the spraying which might cause serious sickness for her new baby. I accepted and they stayed for two months. We enjoyed our suddenly increased family.

Why must malathion air spraying be applied?

The story goes back to June of 1980 – probably the result of a tourist smuggling a tropical fruit through agricultural inspection in Hawaii – when the fruit fly first appeared in Santa Clara County, located about fifty miles south of San Francisco.

By January, the insect had infested some five-hundred square miles around the county. Governor Brown, trying to control the medfly from the ground, ordered a full-scale ground attack on January 6th. Thousands of state and federal employees and volunteers began a door-to-door campaign, entering infected area backyards carrying rakes and plastic bags and picking any fruit, from avocados to oranges. After that they sprayed malathion insecticide from the ground. Furthermore, California officials imported millions of male medflies from Peru and sterilized them by radiation; they were released to mate with females and produce unfertilized eggs.

However, about six months later they found that many of the males were fertile. Learning that the medfly in California was increasing its numbers and damages, U.S. Agriculture Secretary John Block warned that he would embargo the out-of-state shipment of fruits and vegetables produced by California's $14 billion agricultural industry.

Two hours after the warning on July 10th, Governor Brown permitted aerial spraying of malathion.

Since then, about three months have passed. The environmentalists could not successfully oppose aerial spraying to kill the medfly, risking possible human sickness, because everybody knows the medfly would destroy California's billion-dollar industry without it. Therefore, aerial spray of malathion is continuing. Now, six more counties have started spraying, including the Central Valley area. Are we winning the war against the medfly? It seems to me the answer is no. On October 9th, TV news reported that about forty-five medfly eggs were found on fruit in Alameda County.

What is the medfly?

The medfly is one of the fruit fly family and it is the most dreaded among the fruit flies. It has long been a pest in Africa, Australia, South America, and on the Hawaiian and Bermuda Islands, destroying peaches, apricots, pears, oranges, tangerines, and other cultivated fruits. Its name is misleading because the fly was introduced into the Mediterranean area relatively recently. Being the size of a rice grain, smaller than a regular house fly, and with yellow stripes on its wings, the medfly is quite beautiful. However, for fruit farmers, it is enemy number one. According to Masanobu Fukuoka, a Japanese natural farming agriculturist and philosopher, the

medfly is the most fearful attacker for fruits because once its
eggs are laid (sometimes five hundred at a time), the larvae
tunnel into the fruit and make it unfit for human consumption
by turning the flesh of the fruit into a brown viscous mass.
According to *Business Week*, January 19, 1981, it will damage
250 kinds of fruit and vegetables – including oranges, plums,
apples, apricots, tomatoes, eggplants, and so on. The medfly
appeared in Florida in 1956; by heavy aerial spray, it was
eradicated in 1957. Due to strong resistance against all insecticides and the potentiality of damage to fruits, worldwide quarantine laws were formed at that time to regulate the entry of
fruits into other countries.

At present, continents which are not infested by the medfly
are North America and Asia. All other continents are. Therefore, America prohibits importing fruits from Europe, the
Near East, Africa, Australia, and Brazil. If the U.S. fails to
control the medfly, Japan will be infested soon. Japan has been
importing almost a billion dollars worth of fruit from California per year. Even the quarantine will not be able to stop a
medfly invasion, because some innocent fruit lover or greedy
merchants will smuggle fruits and medflies into Japan. Then
the medfly will invade Korea and China, to complete the world
invasion.

In order to stop the medfly invasion, California used two
tactics. One was an insecticide spray and the other was a
quarantine. Of course these are not the best remedies. Officials
used these tactics only because there were no other tactics they
could find. We had a report from a friend who lives in the
spraying area. She reported to us, "The prevalent attitude here
seems to be this spray is something we don't like but that we
must live with it, adapt our lives around it." According to her,
"Many people are complaining of sore throats, coughs, and
colds but tend to blame this on the weather becoming colder
and windier. A nurse at a local hospital said she thought that

any number of health complaints could be an outcome of contact with the spray. This is contrary to the standard statement given out by the medfly information office – they insist the only reaction to the organo-phosphates would be headache and nausea."

According to *Assessment of the Health Risks from the Proposed Aerial Application of Malathion*, prepared by the California Department of Health Services, December 1980, the risk, using the most conservative assumption and an extreme worst case example, is one in a million that an exposed child would develop cancer as a result of its exposure to malathion. This figure is probably right, but the problem is that there are so many cancer risks in our present society – x-ray, chemical colorings, preservatives, food conditioners, chemical fertilizers, synthetic feeds, hormone feeds, water and air pollution – that while the risk of each may be one out of a million, when these are added up, one out of a million may end up one out of hundreds or tens. This is one of the reasons that there is one cancer victim out of every four people, according to recent statistics. Even if we do not count cancer risks, there are other health hazards caused by malathion spray.

A similar thought (cumulative toxicity) was expressed twenty years ago by Rachel Carson in *Silent Spring* (Houghton Mifflin Co., 1962):

> A few years ago a team of Food and Drug Administration scientists discovered that when malathion and certain other organic phosphates are administered simultaneously a massive poisoning results – up to 50 times as severe as would be predicted on the basis of adding together the toxicities of the two. In other words, 1/100 of the lethal dose of each compound may be fatal when the two are combined.
>
> This discovery led to the testing of other combinations. It is now known that many pairs of organic phosphate insecticides are highly dangerous, the toxicity

being stepped up or 'potentiated' through the combined action. The two need not be given simultaneously. The hazard exists not only for the man who may
spray this week with one insecticide and next week with
another; it exists also for the consumer of sprayed products. The common salad bowl may easily present a
combination of organic phosphate insecticides.

The toxicity of an organic phosphate can be increased
by a second agent that is not necessarily an insecticide.
For example, one of the plasticizing agents may act even
more strongly than another insecticide to make malathion more dangerous. Again, this is because it inhibits
the liver enzyme that normally would 'draw the teeth' of
the poisonous insecticide.

It seems to me that malathion is less toxic compared to other
pesticides even though it is not completely safe. However, the
trouble is not its toxicity but its effectiveness. Malathion spray
does not completely eradicate the medfly; also, it increases its
resistance. Therefore, several months after spraying, the
medfly often comes back. Probably before we kill the medfly
completely by spray, we will kill the human race unless we find
a better way.

Another protection is the quarantine, which is a more yin
method than the insecticide spray because it tries to exclude
fruits coming from the infected area. This creates financial and
political problems instead of health problems. Before the aerial
spray started this summer, the Japanese government stopped
purchase of California fruits from the infected area due to
possible contamination by medfly maggots or eggs. This will
cause almost a billion-dollar loss to California farmers. The
problems do not stop here. Political problems develop. One
California assemblyman said the State of California should
boycott Japanese goods. He didn't understand the reason
Japan stopped the purchase of California fruits. Probably he
didn't want to understand but rather wanted to try to solve the

problem politically. Such a solution will make the situation worse.

In September three Japanese agricultural officers were invited to the Santa Clara area; they made a recommendation to the Japanese government that fruit importation be permitted. On October 10th the first Sunkist oranges arrived in Japan after the reopening of fruit trade from California.

The California farmers were happy, thinking they had solved at least one of the problems caused by the medfly. However, superficial solutions such as spraying insecticide always bring other problems. Tokyo UPI reported on Saturday, October 10th:

> Japanese longshoremen Friday refused to handle a shipload of California fruit sprayed with toxic insecticide declared cancer-causing in the United States. Chairman Kaneo Hanada of the Yokohama Longshoreman's Union said the workers had unloaded eleven containers of California oranges and other fruits brought in by the 25,000-ton Sealand Liberator.
>
> "But we will not open the containers or move them out from the yard until health officials prove that the fruits or their containers were not stained by the toxic ethylene dibromide (EDB) gas," he said.
>
> The load was the first cargo of fruit sterilized with the EDB gas since the discovery of Mediterranean fruit flies in California.
>
> The Japanese government agreed with U.S. agriculture officials September 8th on EDB sterilization of California oranges, lemons, grapefruit, grapes, and avocados picked outside the medfly contaminated areas for export to Japan. But U.S. Environmental Protection Agency experiments on animals have discovered the EDB could cause cancer and liver trouble. The agency plans to ban EDB beginning in 1983 for that reason.
>
> "It is not fair to use this type of insecticide, which has been found to be dangerous in the United States, on

fruit shipped to Japan," Hanada said. . . .
   A 30,000 ton containership, the Queen's Way Bridge,
is scheduled to dock at Kobe with eighty-six tons of
oranges and seventeen tons of lemons.

Nobody knows how this problem will be solved. I imagine
that the Japanese official who negotiated with U.S. agricultural officials and gave permission to ship California fruits with
EDB spray would resign his job in order to show he failed to
perform his responsibility, which is to protect the Japanese
people from bad fruits. He yielded to the claim of American
scientists and farmers that California fruits are absolutely safe
for Japanese agriculture. But he didn't think whether California fruits are safe for the Japanese people. Therefore, the
question is which is more important - people's health, or the
farmer's income.
   Governor Brown took the stand of people's health first, then
finally yielded to the farmers. The Japanese officer took the
second stand first - protection of Japanese farmers. However,
a big problem is now faced: union protestation and boycott.
   Insecticide and the quarantine cannot solve this dualistic
problem - that is to say, whether people's health or the
farmer's income is more important.
   From the macrobiotic viewpoint, I suggest the following
solution.
   Change farming methods so that the medfly or other insects
do not seriously damage crops grown without insecticide
spray. Giving much fertilizer, especially chemical ones, makes
plants and fruits weaker and more yin (usually yin manifests as
bigger, juicier, and sweeter; therefore, farmers as well as consumers like this type). As a result, fruits are damaged easily by
flies or insects. This is the manifestation of natural selection.
However, if fruits are grown without fertilizer, tilling, insecticide, and weeding, as with Mr. Fukuoka's natural farming,

then plants grow naturally and fit the environment very well. The fruits will be very yang. This means they will not be easily attacked or colonized by fruit flies. Fruit flies don't like yang fruits – they prefer yin ones which are very juicy and sweet.

According to Mr. Fukuoka, if we do natural farming, we do not need insecticide.

Natural farming is the ideal method for any type of agriculture; however, it will not be realized soon. Therefore we need another tactic.

In 1977 the American government published the *U.S. Dietary Goals*, recommending the reduction of animal foods consumption. However, if we only reduce animal foods consumption, we may cause imbalance in our diet.

Animal foods are strong acid forming foods and contain much protein, fat, and sodium. Contrary to animal foods, fruits are strong alkaline forming foods and contain much fruit sugar, vitamins, and potassium. Therefore, animal foods in the diet are well balanced with fruits as dessert. However, if animal food consumption is reduced as recommended in the *Dietary Goals*, then the consumption of fruit must also be reduced; without animal foods, overconsumption of fruits will result in a yin condition caused by too much fruit sugar and vitamins. (Yin symptoms are coldness, tiredness, obesity, various inflammations, loss of menstruation, anemic conditions, frigidity, etc.)

Let us encourage farmers to change from fruit farming to grain farming. This makes grain less expensive and people will eat more grain in their diet which will improve their health. If the price of grain goes down, grain farmers will face a decreased income. To compensate for this drawback, we could create a fruit production tax and give this revenue to grain growers. Higher tax will increase the price of fruit and this will discourage people's overconsumption of fruit. Also, in order to succeed in reducing fruit farming, the United States government must educate the public that fruit consumption can be reduced to one to two pounds a week per person.

If people eat less fruit and eat more grain, the farmers will grow less fruit and more grain. Then the medfly spray will be unnecessary. This is the real solution to the medfly syndrome.

March 1982

America Learns From Japan

I

On December 7, 1941, more than forty years ago, Japanese navy planes attacked Pearl Harbor in order to break the blockade of her oil import route from Indonesia. Before this, Japan joined the Rome-Berlin Axis and finally declared war against the Allies in order to survive their death threat. Due to the war strategy taught by the ancient Chinese strategist Son Tse, the Japanese military government decided to attack Pearl Harbor before the Americans were ready. This action shook the American people, American industries, and the government – leading to the atomic bombing of Hiroshima and Nagasaki four years later which killed 313,814 women, children, and unarmed civilians. This caused the Japanese government to offer a complete surrender; by this surrender Japan lost all her investments and claims in Manchuria, Formosa, Okinawa, and Karafuto. Almost 75 million people were forced to live on an island smaller than California which produced only a little oil, coal, iron and other metals, and timber. It produced no wool, cotton, livestock, milk, etc. What Japan could produce enough for her needs were rice and fish and vegetables. This could sustain health with the consumption of whole grains and vegetables without processing and chemicals.

When the war ended on August 15, 1945, most of the large

cities of Japan were ruined. Houses, schools, hospitals, factories, stores, offices, industries, and communication and transportation systems were shut down. The government issued rationed foods: white rice, sweet potatoes, and soybeans. According to Paul Langer's *Japan: Yesterday and Today* (Holt, Rinehart, and Winston, Inc., 1966), "During the first year after the war, the daily per capita food consumption in Tokyo dropped to 1300 calories, compared with 2200 in the 1930s and over 3000 for the average American. The growing food shortage in the urban areas was further intensified by lack of transportation and fuel. This made it difficult to supply the cities with food and prevented fishing boats from putting out to sea. In order to survive, the city people by the thousands ventured into the countryside daily, where they sought to barter clothing and other belongings for food." In other words, those who had no jobs took the train, went to the farmers, and exchanged their clothing or other goods for potatoes, rice and vegetables, miso and soy sauce, etc., at black market prices; they then came back to town and sold to the rich at a good profit. They were sometimes caught by police who were checking at the stations. The policemen took the foods from these poor carriers (we called them *yamishi*) and kept them for themselves and their families as an extra bonus.

About a quarter of the nation's wealth had been destroyed by the air raid. Japan lacked everything including housing, clothing, and fuel. Food especially was so scarce that people were crazy for foods for at least six months. Farmers sold their produce at extra high prices; after the war many farmers became rich, having introduced mechanized agriculture and the production of more foods. The postwar economy of Japan began its recovery through the farmers.

At that time, commodities needed by the people were thankfully released from army and navy surplus goods by the U.S. occupation authorities. In 1945, 72.4 million Japanese had to be fed. Japan imported about a million dollars worth of food daily from America until 1950 (*Japan: Yesterday and Today*). Rice, wheat, soybeans, etc., were the main commodities.

What the Japanese needed were not only foods but everything else used in daily living such as house- and kitchenwares, clothing, hardware, bicycles, carts, cars and trucks, etc. At my father's factory, a metalworks forge, his workers made iron pans; one day I took them and sold them on the street. They sold like hotcakes. Anything sold, instantly, because everything was destroyed by the bombing. Gradually the streets were cleaned and stores were reopened. Many factories started operating again. As more people returned from evacuation places in the countryside, transportation vehicles were needed. Motorcycles started being manufactured again, and cars followed. Honda, Nissan, and Toyota were such companies. They started from scratch – probably with $500 initial capital, as each company was limited to this as starting capital. It was amazing to see Toyota and Nissan reaching over $13 billion in sales in 1980.

In 1963, Japanese auto manufacturers exported only 7500 passenger cars and trucks, worth about $7 million, to the United States (*The American Automobile,* John B. Rae, University of Chicago Press, 1965); in 1980 they exported 2.4 million cars to America, worth $10 billion. Contrarily, American auto manufacturers had their worst sales crisis. The Chrysler Corporation lost $200 million in 1978, $1.1 billion in 1979, and $1.7 billion in 1980. The Ford Company lost $1.5 billion and General Motors lost over $700 million in 1980. In the same year, fifteen American auto factories and sixteen hundred dealerships were closed (*Japanese Business Strategy*, Nomura Institute, Japanese edition, 1981).

Since the American auto industry accounts for 16 to 20 percent of the GNP, the decline of the domestic auto industry is a significant factor in the declining U.S. economy. This is the reason the American government and unions are forcing the Japanese government to regulate Japanese auto export, even though American business is based on the concept of free competition. Finally in 1981 the Japanese government gave in to American force and announced a self-control policy on the exportation of passenger cars. Now Japanese passenger car manufacturers can export only 65.5 percent of their capacity (*Japanese Business Strategy*). However, this was not the solution. The American automobile situation became worse at the end of 1981. On November 9, *Newsweek* reported:

> General Motors Corporation chairman Roger B. Smith called it 'unique for GM, the auto industry and, as far as we know, for any major U.S. manufacturer.' He did not exaggerate. In a ceremony last week in Clark, New Jersey, Smith handed over the deed to GM's Hyatt roller-bearing plant in return for a down payment of $15 million in cash and 100,000 shares of preferred stock. Receiving the deed was Alan V. Lowenstein, representing a group of former GM workers who had raised $60 million, bought the plant and voted to cut their own wages by 25 percent – all for a very compelling reason: to save their jobs.
>
> Until recently, the very idea of giant General Motors selling one of its plants to its employees would have been unthinkable. This is a sign of the sorry times for the auto industry, now in the third year of the worst automotive recession in half a century. Sales in the first 20 days in October took a nose dive, falling 130,480 units below sales for the same period last year. Ford Motor Co. and Chrysler Corp. last week reported third quarter losses of $355 million and $149 million respectively – capping GM's earlier announcement of a $468 million loss.

The American auto industry was so much worse at the beginning of 1982 that UAW president Douglas A. Fraser offered GM chairman Smith a reduction of their labor salaries corresponding to a proposed reduction in retail car prices, in order to help the company compete with Japanese-made cars (*Business Week*, January 25, 1982). This attitude between labor leaders and corporate executives is an indication that American businesses will be forced to reach the kind of cooperation between management and labor forces which Japan has been practicing for years.

Another Japanese industry which has developed so much that the Japanese government had to control product export was the iron and steel industry – even though Japan has to import the raw materials for steel production. Producing 32.9 million tons of iron and steel in 1980, Japanese Shin Nippon Seitetsu K.K. was the world's highest producer, producing more than the total output of either Italy (26.5 million tons) or France (23.1 million tons). Japanese iron and steel companies are leading their once technological teachers, America and Europe, not only in quantity but also in quality. The following are only a few examples: In 1980, Sumitomo Metal Industries exported the large steel tube manufacturing technique to U.S. Steel; in 1981, New Nippon Seitetsu received an order from the Pittsburgh Steel Company to construct a $100 million casting factory; and the Nippon Kokan Company is negotiating with the Ford Motor Company for a merger with its steel production company, Rouge River Steel (*Japanese Business Strategy*).

The Japanese are hard workers but they are not slaves to their jobs. They like to enjoy their lives. They enjoy sports, music, dancing, and all amusements. This is the reason two army engineers began a tape recorder manufacturing company with $500 capital in May of 1946, a year after the Japanese surrender. The streets of Tokyo were still burnt smelling – there was disorder, people were sleeping in shacks made of tin plates, and most stores were closed. These two men, Masaru Ibuka and Akira Morita, knew that the Japanese like entertainments and therefore they felt products such as tape recorders and radios would be good sales items. This company is, of course, Sony Corporation. They purchased the rights to the use of the transistor in 1953 from the Western Electric Company with an advance payment of $25,000. The sum was too high for their financial situation and it was a great gamble for them to spend such big money – but this was the important decision which made Sony a household name all over the world twenty-five years later.

While she failed in attacking Pearl Harbor in 1941, Japan won the North American continent via Japanese products.

When I came to America in 1952, most Japanese goods were considered cheap and were found at the ten-cent stores. Shortly thereafter, Sony's transistor radios and especially their television sets changed this image. Color television sets made by Sony, Matsushita, Hitachi, Toshiba, Sharp, and Sanyo acquired 40 percent of the American market in 1976. They were producing almost twice as many sets as American companies produced in 1975. The importation of Japanese products increased so quickly that some American factories were closed and some 65,000 workers laid off. The American color TV protection committee asked the U.S. government to increase import duty on Japanese sets, but President Carter rejected this. However, the Japanese government, recognizing the American economic situation, offered that the maximum TV set exportation to the U.S. would be 1.75 million per year for a three-year period. This was 41 percent of the Japanese color TV export capacity of that year (*Japanese Business Strategy*).

Japanese exportation of steel, automobiles, televisions, and the transistor created many conflicts in the American economy. However, Japanese motorcycles, cameras, copy machines, pianos, and fasteners (zippers) found no competition in the American market. If America were to manufacture them domestically, Japanese manufacturers would be big competitors.

The amazing Japanese economic power appeared not only in the amount of its exportation but also in its own economic situation. While the U.S. and most European countries are experiencing double-digit inflation and a sluggish economic condition, Japan appears to be the only exception; that is to say, she has single-digit inflation, low interest rates for loans, and high-growth GNP. Japanese companies are distinguished from American and European companies in the following areas: low unemployment ratio, few labor strikes, better corporate profit, and better stock market performance.

II

In America as well as Europe, many scholars and writers have been reporting the amazing economic growth of Japan following World War II. Ezra F. Vogel, professor of sociology at Harvard University, says in his *Japan As No. 1* (Harvard University Press, 1979) that America ought to learn much from Japan. Japan has been learning from Europe and America to improve her systems – she is learning even after having already learned, in order to further improve – but the Americans have never tried to learn from other than European countries, even when they realized their system was not working well. Professor Vogel reasons why the Japanese had such economic success. First of all, they are always trying to accumulate knowledge and information – whether as a business corporation, a union, central or local government, or an individual. For example, there are no American companies that can compete with the amount and accuracy of information accumulated by Japanese trading companies. Secondly, in Japanese business the accumulated knowledge and information are applied to decision-making by group effort. Therefore, decisions are generally the result of careful research and majority support. Thirdly, Japanese businessmen learned business systems from Europe at the beginning of the twentieth century, improving their own. Characteristic in the Japanese system are: long-term planning, lifetime employment with wage increase by age, and loyalty to the company.

The long-term plan: Japanese businesses are based more on future than short-term profit. Because of this, Japanese companies invest in better equipment and research. This type of business operation is possible as they do not depend on public investment but rather on bank loans. Vogel reports that 50 percent of the capital for American companies comes from public investment, while in Japan the figure is only 10 percent. Therefore, Japanese companies can aim towards future profit without pressure from shareholders, who always want profit showing now rather than in the future.

The long-term plan relates closely with **lifetime employment**. In Japan most people stay with one company from school graduation until retirement, which is around the age of fifty-seven. By this system the company offers steady increases in wage, post, and welfare and retirement benefits. The employee has no worries about loss of job unless an unusual recession comes, and in the case of bankruptcy the company arranges new jobs for its employees. Larger companies in Japan are supported by banks and banks are supported by government; therefore, if officers are honest and sincere, companies are hardly ever bankrupt. Since employees work at the same company their whole life, they naturally become loyal. Some feel devotion to the company. This company devotion makes the Japanese business system very unusual – that is to say, it is a 'bottom-up' system. Lower-position workers take the initiative for planning, studying, gathering information, and contacting other workers, and they give advice to their superiors.

Finally, employers and employees of Japanese companies

are united in a **one-family spirit**. This is similar to the American college fraternities. Many big businesses have their own resorts, company dormitories, and even sports teams. American professional athletic teams are owned by individuals, but in Japan they are owned by business companies. Employees are united in spirit by playing sports together.

The Japanese tendency toward groupism runs deep. For example, American workers worry about position and salary because these are the measures of their achievement. For Japanese workers, position and salary are not measurements of achievement. The most important valuation for them is the respect and trust of the other workers. Vogel pointed out that American executives will fire employees in order to continue paying dividends to shareholders. Such an attitude naturally creates labor's distrust of management. Japanese executives will not do such a thing.

Professor Vogel discusses the Japanese system very well in many fields, including government and politics, business, education, social welfare, and crime problems. His observations are surprisingly correct. After such observations he advises us what Americans should learn from Japan. However, he is not a mere admirer of Japan. He is very well aware of Japan's shortcomings, which of course he advises us not to learn.

Another economist who admired the Japanese economic growth and discusses its causes is Peter F. Drucker. He probes Japan's miraculous economic development in his *Men, Ideas, and Politics* (Harper & Row, 1971):

> Japan was almost overrun these few years by Western economists, bankers, and industrialists who had come to study the Japanese economic miracle. Arthur Burns, chairman of the Council of Economic Advisers under Eisenhower, was there in 1963. For instance, he was so impressed, according to reports, that he strongly

recommended that President Kennedy adopt some of Japan's tax and money policies to spur our laggard economy. . . . What has happened in Japan since the end of the American occupation in April 1951 is the most extraordinary success story in all economic history.

Drucker points out the reasons for Japan's success story as follows: First, the Japanese invested more than a quarter of their national income. Second, they created a mass consumer market and a stock market that is the second largest in the world (next to the U.S.) with almost no resources. Third, she has the greatest young collegiate population in the world next only to the U.S. and Israel. Fourth, the modern Japanese lifespan expanded from fifty to seventy, equal to that of the most advanced countries in the West.

In my study of the economic success of Japan, Professor Drucker is the only one I found who has pointed to health conditions as the cause of such success. On this I will discuss more later.

In the economic development of Japan, Drucker considers the following three business systems the most important:

Consensus decision-making.

In *Men, Ideas, and Politics,* he explains why he recommends consensus decision-making: "In the first place, it actually makes for speedy decisions and above all, for effective decisions. It takes a much longer time in Japan to reach a decision than it takes in the West. But we in the West then spend years on selling a decision. We make the decision first and then begin to work on getting people to act on it. And, only too often, as all of us in the West know, either the decision is sabotaged by the organization or, which may be worse, it takes so long to make it truly effective that it has become obsolete."

Lifetime employment.

He admits that the lifetime employment system as it exists in Japanese companies may cause drawbacks: "As a result most Japanese industry is grossly overstaffed, and thousands of people, for whom there are no jobs, are kept on doing almost nothing in the plant or office." It seems to me this is an extreme case and that most Japanese companies are so well managed that there are no persons around plants or offices who have nothing to do. I agree it is sometimes impossible to maintain lifetime employment. (Therefore, another writer, Professor William Ouchi, recommends long-term instead of lifetime employment.) However, Drucker admits this system works better psychologically compared to the Western system of employment: "Economically, it might be said, we have greater security in our system; we certainly pay more for it. Yet we have not obtained what the Japanese system produces: the psychological conviction of lifetime employment, that is, of job and income security."

Youth education.

Young employees who will be the company's future executives are cared for and educated by the company. According to Drucker, Japanese companies have 'godfathers' who educate special young employees so that they can be future executives. He is not sure how this concept can be applied to the American system; however, he sees if this is done it will bring quite a benefit to the American companies as it will eliminate the generation gap in the management of the future company. UCLA's Dr. Ouchi has a similar view on this, discussed later.

English writer P.B. Stone is another admirer of the miraculous development of the postwar Japanese economy. He describes it in the introduction to *Japan Surges Ahead* (Frederick A. Praeger, 1969): "A British working man of twenty-five years of age cannot expect to double his real earnings until he is fifty. A Japanese working man can expect it in seven or eight years – that is what an economic miracle feels like to an ordinary person." In the first chapter he writes, "The extreme paucity of natural resources is a most important feature of Japan. It has been a tremendous handicap and the story of Japan's economic growth is all the more remarkable because of it. If the Japanese had been able to occupy Australia or Alaska – both full of natural resources – it seems probable that the world would have been able to witness an even more remarkable surge of economic development which would, quite possibly, have put the Japanese people on a par with the United States by 1980." However, I don't agree with this opinion. In my opinion, the scarcity of resources in fact caused the miraculous development of Japan's economy. If Japan had resources like the U.S. or China, she would not have developed the famous Japanese trading companies by which she can obtain anything she needs at the cheapest prices and can sell her products anywhere on the globe. For example, the World Trade Building, the highest building in New York City, was constructed of Japanese steel. Why? Because a Japanese trading company could sell cheaper than American manufacturers. The competitive research on the part of these companies results in their ability to buy and sell on the world market at the lowest cost. Often this means that materials are transported to factories by boat instead of train or trucks, and this reduces costs even further; for example, freight cost by boat from New York to Japan is less than from Pittsburgh to New York by truck.

Stone thinks the human factors are the most important causes in Japanese economic development. On this, I agree. However, he misunderstands the Japanese mentality. He writes, ". . . loyalty to Japan herself has been a potent factor in encouraging exports whilst discouraging imports." This is his misunderstanding, as Japan has been a great admirer of foreign goods and cultures. The Japanese are always looking for foreign goods and are proud of their possession. The only reason they can export more than they can import is that their technological development has made it possible. Ten percent of Japan's GNP is spent to import materials from all over the world. She adds brain work, machine work, and manual work to it and produces ten times the worth in final products. Only one-tenth of the value of the final production is exported, so that she can import the raw materials, and nine-tenths of the finished products are kept for her own use. Therefore, Japan is not a competitive exporter but rather she is an importer. In 1974 Japan's exports, at 9.8 percent of the GNP, were less than those of France (12.3 percent), the United Kingdom (16.6 percent), or West Germany (18.8 percent) – less than any major nation except America (4.4 percent) and the U.S.S.R. (*Japan Today*, William H. Forbes, Harper, 1975).

Two current bestsellers deal with Japan's economic success. One is *The Art of Japanese Management* (Simon and Schuster, 1981) by Richard Pascal, lecturer in business administration at Stanford's Graduate School of Business, and Anthony G. Athos, professor of the school of business at Harvard. The other is *Theory Z* (Addison Wesley Publishing Co., 1981) by William Ouchi, professor of business administration at UCLA's Graduate School of Business. Both are very well written and original books.

"There is a disturbing tendency in America to focus on some of the more exotic features of Japanese methods, such as company songs, morning calisthenics, and lifetime employment," Pascal writes. "These exist, but they are by no means the main reasons why the Japanese are successful. Many of their successes are entirely attributable to their having a superior marketing strategy. For example, the Japanese tried to introduce their motorcycles in the U.S. through the usual dealer networks, but they were laughed out of the Harley-Davidson shops. So they decided to form their own dealerships and their own market plan.

"They pioneered the leisure class market and changed the entire nature of the motorcycle business. No longer are motorcycles just sold to the leather jacket-clad. The example is significant because Honda's success had nothing to do with the company songs or lifetime employment. They simply outsmarted us."

In *Theory Z*, Professor Ouchi compares systems between Japanese and American business companies. He cites lifetime employment, slow promotion, the non-specialization career course, and decision-making by group as the reasons why Japanese businesses developed so well. He also realizes Japanese-type organizations already exist in America. He calls them Z-type organizations. According to him, Z-type organizations employ the above systems, except 'lifetime employment' is changed to 'long-term'. He explains why these systems are important. Long-term employment creates trust among employees and employers. Employees accept slow promotion and the non-specialization career course because they know they will be able to work a long time for the company. This avoids competitive attitudes among employees; instead, they help each other. Decision-making by group, according to Professor Ouchi, creates a willingness to work on the part of the employees much more than with the individual decision-making style. The plan decided by group will be easily supported by all, while the plan decided by a few will face difficulties in achieving agreement later. Such are some of the characteristics of Z-type organizations. According to Ouchi, General Motors, IBM, Hewlett-Packard, Rockwell International, Intel, and Procter & Gamble are examples of Z-type organizations.

Characteristic of Professor Ouchi's approach is his thinking that psychological improvement is more essential than mechanical or structural improvement of the management in order to achieve a Z-type organization. In other words, the well-organized, profitable Z-type organization should have mutual trust, thoughtfulness, and intimacy among all workers – including executives. Such an organization will create humanistic working conditions in the company instead of a cold, mechanical, and inhumane working place. If people work with more intimacy, Ouchi thinks, the American divorce rate will be reduced. With the lack of intimacy in the workplace, people cannot talk to co-workers about such things as family difficulties. Then the husband and wife will complain to each other when they come home from work, certainly bringing no joy to either. Such a family tends to break up. When the family situation is not good it is natural that people cannot work well at their jobs. Ouchi's advice for improving American business can be seen in the improvement of 'softwares' while Dr. Vogel's approach improves 'hardwares'.

III

The economic success of Japan depends on a distinctive management style, which I have introduced through various Western writers and economists. In my opinion, they are mostly correct, although some Japanese social behavior is not in my favor – such as the tendency to be too concerned with relationships and with social recognition. In any case, in order to succeed economically, Japan created a distinguished business style which in the final analysis is a creation of the Japanese way of thinking. What is the Japanese way of thinking that created such a miraculous economic surge after World War II?

One of these ways of thinking is the attitude toward work. Mitsuko Shimomura writes on this in the November, 1981 issue of *Science Digest*.

> I have felt that the difference between Eastern and Western management is rooted in attitudes toward work. In general, people of the Western countries see work as a restriction on personal liberty; one trades freedom for a salary. Managers don't trust workers to further the interests of the company, and workers feel used by their firms.
>
> In Japan, however, work is not considered to be an infringement on human freedom. The Japanese believe that to work is to live and that at work one establishes one's identity. Neither blue- nor white-collar workers consider their interests to be opposed to those of the company; a worker's salary and bonuses reflect the company's success.

Another Japanese way of thinking which is quite influential in the Japanese business style is their order of thinking. For example, in writing an address the Japanese begin with the country's name, then the town, street, and finally the individual's name. Contrary to this, Westerners write their addresses starting with the individual's name and ending with the country. When we live on different planets in the future, Westerners will end their address with the name of the planet while the Japanese will start the address with it. I call the Japanese approach the 'centripetal way of thinking'. This means one's order of thinking goes from outside to inside, or large to small, or ultimate to immediate. This is shown in the example of the address. I call the Western way of thinking the 'centrifugal way' – that is to say, it begins by dealing with small things or details and then tries to reach large general laws or conclusions. Physics, for example, begins with the smallest living units. Science is the result of centrifugal thinking, and therefore it is natural that science developed in the West. On the other hand, religion and philosophy developed in the East through contemplation of the ultimate, or nature, on the part of wise men. The Japanese are accustomed to this kind of centripetal thinking in which one begins from general laws and ends up with individual cases. Science is limited by physical observation and the senses, while religion and philosophy tend to be dogmatic.

Most Japanese have been familiar with the centripetal way of thinking – religious and philosophical thought. This Japanese way of thinking – the centripetal way, or it may be called groupism – grew under the longtime influence of Shinto and Buddhism. However, after contact with Western culture following the signing of the Kanagawa Treaty on March 31, 1854, the Japanese acquired much of the Western way of thinking also. They achieved a mingling of Eastern and Western thinking. This is one of the most important causes for Japan having risen from nowhere to third in the World in economic development within a hundred years. Although they have learned the Western way of individualistic thinking very well, the Japanese still maintain the Eastern mentality deep in their thinking. For this reason the Japanese consider their nation, society, family, and group more important than the individual. Edwin O. Reischauer writes in *The Japanese* (Harvard University Press, 1979):

> Certainly no difference is more significant between Japanese and American, or Westerners in general, than the greater Japanese tendency to emphasize the group, somewhat at the expense of the individual. . . . The Japanese are much more likely than Westerners to operate in groups or at least to see themselves as operating in this way. Where Westerners may at least put on a show of independence and individuality, most Japanese will be quite content to conform in dress, conduct, style of life, and even thought to the norms of their group.

Due to this kind of thinking, the company they work for is not just a mere employer but is their source of bread and butter.

They respect the employer and are loyal to the company. The company executives, in return, respond to this loyalty and try to keep workers until retirement by all means. Thus, Japanese business created the systems of the long-term plan, lifetime employment, wage increase by age, etc., at which many Western economists and businessmen are awed.

An October 19, 1981 article in *Time* magazine by John Leo entitled "Samurai Killing on the Market" reported that the Japanese samurai Miyamoto Musashi's book had become a bestseller in the business world of New York City. This happened, according to the article, because advertising executive George Lois wrote in *Adweek* magazine that "the Japanese entrepreneur is not nurtured at an Asian equivalent of our Harvard Business School. Instead, he studies, lives and works according to an almost mythic tome written in 1645 by the great samurai, Miyamoto Musashi . . . the classic *A Book of Five Rings*" (translated by Victor Harris, The Overlook Press, 1974).

I am sure that most readers of this English translation will not understand the meaning of Musashi's last chapter, Ku, or Nothingness. This chapter explains his philosophical view of oneness. Musashi struggled to achieve the mastery of swordsmanship and after fighting over sixty times without losing, in deep contemplation he reached the concept of oneness. He says in this chapter that the aim of swordsmanship is to understand oneness, where no enemy exists and where fighting is not necessary. One who does not understand this last chapter will wholly misunderstand Musashi's greatness, as well as the Japanese mentality. That is to say, for the Japanese, oneness is most important, and the individual is a part of the One.

The next thing I believe to be an important cause of the Japanese economic surge is their condition of good health maintained after World War II when compared with European and American countries. This fact is well documented by statistics in *The Book of Numbers* (edited by Heron House Publishing, LTD, A & W Publishers, 1978):

- 13 percent of the American population in 1977 suffered headaches regularly while this was the case in only 0.47 percent of the Japanese population.

- In 1976, 540,000 Americans were addicted to narcotics and 92,600 abused drugs (aspirin, barbiturates, tranquilizers, and illegal drugs) while Japanese narcotics addicts numbered 6,400 and drug abuses were at 9,700. Japanese addiction was only 1 percent of the American figure, even though Japan's population is half that of the United States.

- Death from heart disease per 100,000 in America was 338.2 but 109.1 in Japan in 1976.

- Death from cancer in America was more than double that of Japan in 1974.

- The most terrifying comparison is with mental retardation; 30.4 out of 10,000 Americans were admitted to mental hospitals during 1970 while this was only 13.2 in Japan. The same year, 63.3 out of 10,000 Americans were diagnosed with mental illness; however, this number increased to 104.2 per 10,000 in 1974. One out of every 100 Americans were mentally ill.

When we study these statistics, it seems obvious why American business and the economy went downward while the Japanese economy increased.

What made the difference in health as it appeared in the statistics between Japan and America, in my opinion, is their differences in diet. This has been mentioned by some scientists and U.S. government officers. In this article I do not intend to discuss this subject at length. Those interested in further study might read the relevant health literature. However, I would like to say that the Japanese diet, which in fact is close to the recommendations of the Senate Select Committee on Nutrition in 1977, is one of the most important factors in Japan's successful economic development.

Since the traditional Japanese diet has been Americanized more recently, their health is declining. Therefore, their success in business will not last unless they change their diet back again.

IV

Once American workers acquire company loyalty as in the case of Japanese workers, the quality of production, enthusiasm toward work, quality control, and long-term employment will be improved as seen in the Japanese companies. In my opinion, executives of the huge American corporations overlook the fact that human nature at large is the same, East or West. Loyalty among Japanese workers to their companies is actually competitiveness existing between similar companies. Two of the largest trading companies in Japan, Mitsui and Mitsubishi, have been competitors for over a hundred years. This competitiveness makes workers loyal to their companies.

This is the same mentality as, for example, when UCLA or USC students are loyal to their respective football teams. Without football games between UCLA and USC, loyalty among the students would not be built. It is the same for cities. San Franciscans or Northern Californians are loyal fans of the 49ers; Los Angeles people are loyal to the Rams. Once this loyalty to one team is established, it stays with the fans wherever they go. One of my friends is a fan of the Philadelphia Eagles, even when he is living in Northern California. One who grew up in Texas will follow the Dallas Cowboys, of course.

The Japanese use this sentiment or emotional attitude for stimulating the loyalty of workers: that is to say, professional Japanese baseball teams (Japan has no football teams) are owned by businesses or manufacturing companies. Most famous among the professional teams is the Tokyo Giants, named after the San Francisco Giants which were then still playing in New York City. Being one of the strongest teams in Japan and located in the world's most populated city, the Tokyo Giants are the most popular. Its fans are not only the employees of the owner company, Yomiuri News Publishing Company, but also people living in Tokyo as well as suburban areas. Watching games from the stands or on television, they all become friends due to a common denominator – everyone is a fan of the same team. Tokyo citizens are proud of having the great team in their hometown, and company workers are proud supporters of their heroes. Games are the company's social events, and teams are their mascots and symbols.

This system should be brought into the top American manufacturing companies such as General Motors, Ford, Chrysler, U.S. Steel, Arco, Shell, Standard, Exxon, etc. These companies should form their own football or baseball teams and fight toward an Inter-Industries Super Bowl. This way, professional and amateur sports would benefit American industry and economy instead of only a few individual owners. And large corporations would obtain much publicity by owning a team.

Remember how many people became patriotic when the young underdog American hockey team beat the undefeated Russian team in the 1980 Winter Olympics. Likewise, company sport teams would be instrumental in cultivating loyal groupism among workers. In my opinion, Japan's advantage over America in business arises from only one factor: that the Japanese have a better grouping sense, not only between union members but between employers and employees. Creating competitive sports teams would cultivate group bonding and loyalty among workers. This is what American workers and manufacturers need most now.

On January 24, 1982 the San Francisco 49ers won the Super Bowl Championship over the Cincinnati Bengals. Over 500,000 excited fans welcomed the players in downtown San Francisco the following evening. A celebration with over half a million people in a town with a population of about 600,000 is really something. This has not been done for any movie star or rock musician; it was said that this kind of excitement never happened before in San Francisco. In other words, winning a game of sport can excite people as much as winning a war.

In the January 26, 1982 edition of the *San Francisco Chronicle*, Randy Shilts wrote:

> Urban sociologists and business leaders predicted yesterday that the long-term effects of the 49ers Super Bowl victory will include soaring tourism, a stronger sense of community and a better national image for San Francisco.
>
> Richard LeGates, associate professor of Urban Studies at San Francisco State University, said, ". . . the many photographs of blacks and whites, straights and gays, Latinos and Chinese-Americans all jubilantly hugging and chanting together are a major sign of revitalized unity in the city."
>
> E. Barbara Phillips, a sociologist at San Francisco State University, compared the Super Bowl mania to the national uplift that surrounded the release of the U. S. hostages in Iran last year.
>
> At the San Francisco Suicide Prevention Center, executive director Dorothy Stapp said that the numbers of suicide callers dropped by 50 percent after the 49ers' Super Bowl victory. ". . . This tends to happen when people are united around a common social event that's very absorbing and exciting," said Stapp. "People feel a sense of being part of something, a connectedness."

The above report from the San Francisco scene will tell us how much the company sport teams would unite company workers. This would be maintained even when the team is losing, because losing is the beginning of winning. In any event, the greatest benefit the companies would receive by having teams would be increased intimacy between workers and non-workers, including executives, related to the company.

V

My teacher, George Ohsawa, predicted America's economic decline twenty years ago. He wrote in *Zen Macrobiotics* (Ohsawa Foundation, 1965), "The American World Empire (the Gold Dynasty), the monumental achievement of modern civilization, is in the agonies of its death. This finale seems to be the fatal destiny of humanity, for it is occurring for the 25th time in the history of the world. It derives from man's formally logical, analytical, microscopic, mechanical, anatomical, and scientific conception of the universe."

Then Ohsawa offers a gift from the East – something he calls the 'unique principle' and its dietary application, the macrobiotic diet.

> At this crucial time, it is our duty to offer to the American people the greatest gift that we have in the Orient – a supreme, invisible, and ancestral treasure that is 5000 years old. Since we have owed much to Western civilization from the time of Admiral Perry's first visit to Japan one hundred years ago, our gift is offered as a partial payment of that debt. Humbly but with all confidence, we present the 'unique principle' of freedom, health, happiness, and world peace; it will be very useful and informative for our American friends.
>
> The 'unique principle' (the principle of yin and yang) was developed through our ancient philosophy. As

> compared to Western philosophy and science and tech-
> nology which are deterministic, materialistic, analyti-
> cal, anatomical, and atomic, our viewpoint is paradoxi-
> cal, dialectical, panoramic, and universal – a system of
> all-embracing, unificative, and creative contempla-
> tion. . . . The introduction into the Occident of this old
> theory of the Orient will be very interesting. Its biologi-
> cal and physiological technique – macrobiotics – is the
> application of that theory to the art of longevity and
> rejuvenation. It can change Western life completely.
> Here is the 'meeting of East and West' that can produce
> a distinguished new civilization.

Thousands and thousands of Europeans and Americans have observed the macrobiotic diet and way of life. They have improved their health and happiness tremendously. This macrobiotic philosophy and diet is the real cause of Japan's economic success, even though – because their diet has been distant from macrobiotics for awhile – they are not aware of it. This was the original diet in Japan prior to the importation of Western ways, and the Japanese also pretty much returned to this diet for a short while just following World War II due to the food shortage.

From my twenty years of teaching experience in this country, I am convinced that America could be one of the greatest countries in the world if Americans would learn macrobiotics – its diet and philosophy. I agree with George Ohsawa when he said, "Were American understanding of the Oriental mentality and philosophy to be deepened, and were Mortimer Adler (compiler of the *Syntopicon*) to compile another encyclopedia that encompassed Oriental thought, there would no longer be any source for future wars; a new civilization could continue for at least two thousand years."

May 1982

Mother's Education

There are two kinds of education. One is a materialistic education and the other is a spiritual education. The materialistic education is the common school education which is trying to offer knowledge of all science, technology, culture, and art and the techniques of art, crafts, and industry. Since happiness for most people is getting what one wants and the realization of material comfort, materialistic or modern education aims to achieve such happiness through materialistic means and the accumulation of matter called money.

Some will say that the common education aims towards spiritual education also. That is true; however, the majority of education today is materialistic because it gives knowledge and techniques concerning material happiness and comfort. Of course material happiness and comfort are important factors for our total happiness. However, they are not absolute, but relative. In other words, they will change to unhappiness and discomfort sooner or later. And, too, one's happiness may be another's unhappiness. Therefore, materialistic education aims at the majority's happiness but not everyone's and aims at the temporal happiness but not the eternal one.

The spiritual education is the education of absolute and eternal happiness. This kind of education is very hard to give, and one rarely receives it. Those who received this kind of education have always become the great people of man's history.

Since our spirit or virtue manifests through our body, our physical condition is therefore an important factor in spiritual growth. Thus a new education started – macrobiotic education. Macrobiotic education aims towards eternal happiness as well as materialistic comfort and happiness. Macrobiotic education also can be divided in two. The materialistic one teaches macrobiotic knowledge and techniques – selection of foods, cooking, how to eat, prevention and treatment of sicknesses – and explains all phenomena and science through the yin yang wholistic principle and the order of the universe. The other one is the macrobiotic spiritual education. The macrobiotic spiritual education and other spiritual educations are the same because there is only one spiritual education.

What, then, is the spiritual education? The spiritual education is one that teaches us supreme judgment such as absolute honesty, gratefulness without complaint, no exclusivity, no hatred, and no resentment.

How and who can give such an education?

In man's history, great spiritual educators often appeared and taught us supreme judgment. Some were Christ, Buddha, Lao Tsu, and more recently Bab and Baha'u'llah of the Bahai religion. How did they learn the supreme judgment? Were they born with these virtues? In reality everyone has seeds of these virtues. Everybody has the potential to become such a spiritual leader. However, few of us realize supreme judgment and virtues; these are the result of a spiritual education. Then who gave them such education, when they never went to high school or college? Probably they didn't even go to elementary school.

The educator was their mother. The greatest spiritual educator in the world has been and always will be one's mother, who may not have graduated from any college or high school. One mother couldn't even read or write and yet made her son a great man.

Abraham Lincoln, the sixteenth president of the United States, once told his friend Billy Herndon, "All that I am or even hope to be I get from my mother, God bless her." What Lincoln said was almost unbelievable because when his mother, Nancy Hanks, died he was only nine years old. How can a nine-year-old boy learn the virtue or judgment which made him president of the United States as well as one of the most distinguished politicians in human history? Lincoln's formal education was less than one year. Afterwards, he studied by himself with the help of his mother for about three years until she died. Lincoln must have learned his humanity and high judgment – that is to say, his sincerity, integrity, humanistic love, and courage – in this short time. How could his mother teach him such virtues and high judgment in such a short time? This is an example of the spiritual education which is given without words or schoolings. This is the mother's education. She teaches by showing examples and with few words.

Mahatma Gandhi, a spiritual leader of not only India but also the world, lived with his mother just until he was eighteen. When he returned home from London his mother had gone already. Therefore, what he learned from his mother must have been before the age of eighteen. The most important thing he learned from his mother was her saintliness. He said in his autobiography, "The outstanding impression my mother has left on my memory is that of saintliness." He learned his mother's saintliness so well that he was called Mahatma ('soul') by the Indians.

Another thing he learned from his mother was her fasting. What made Gandhi a most distinguished and remarkable revolutionary was his nonviolent leadership. The nonviolent leader's weapon was fasting, by which Gandhi fought Great Britain, united the people of India, and led 400 million Indians to independence. The longest he fasted was over sixty days. He knew how to fast without death. He knew fasting makes the will strong, makes the spirit high, and unites people. Fasting was the only weapon Gandhi used. He learned it from his mother without words when he was still young. He wrote in his *Autobiography: The Story of my Experiments with Truth* (Beacon Press, 1957):

> She was deeply religious. She would not think of taking her meals without her daily prayers. I do not remember her having ever missed the Chaturmas (a vow of fasting and semi-fasting during the four months of the rains). She would take the hardest vows and keep them without flinching. To keep two or three consecutive fasts was nothing to her. Living on one meal a day during Chaturmas was a habit with her. During another Chaturmas she vowed not to have food without seeing the sun. We children on those days would stand, staring at the sky, waiting to announce the appearance of the sun to our mother. And I remember days when, at his sudden appearance, we would rush and announce it to her. She would run out to see with her own eyes, but by that time the fugitive sun would be gone, thus depriving her of her meal. "That does not matter," she would say cheerfully, "God did not want me to eat today." And then she would return to her round of duties.

Thus his mother taught him to fast as well as to not break promises and not lie on any occasion.

Another example of mother's education was told by George Ohsawa, founder of the macrobiotic movement in Western countries. One day in Tokyo around 1963, Ohsawa told us at his seminar about his mother as his lifelong educator:

> My mother was divorced from my father when she was twenty-five, after five years of marriage. Then she studied nursing and midwifery at the Do-Shi-Sha University (a Christian university in Kyoto) in order to support her family. After graduating, she was busy helping

the sick and poor. She was always working hard for the poor. Thus her attitude made me work hard for the sick and poor later. However, within her character the most important thing was that she never complained of sickness, her husband's lack of integrity, financial difficulties, etc. After five years of hard work she contracted tuberculosis, probably due to her bad diet learned from Western nutritional theory (not knowing the macrobiotic diet). When the sickness was very advanced, she called her two surviving sons to her bedside. She told me to become a scholar because I was yin, and my younger brother she told to become a soldier because he was quite yang. After telling us about our future, she lay in bed quietly about thirty minutes and died. She never cried or complained even though she worried about the future of her two sons, resented my father's unfaithful conduct, and was concerned about the family's poor financial situation. This is the education. People often talk too much. Then they cannot impress lifelong virtues or attitudes. My mother taught me 'Do not complain' without words when she was dying. Therefore, I followed it for sixty years and by this virtue I could change thousands of people to macrobiotics. What I am now and want to be in the future is influenced by my mother who died when I was ten.

Thus Lincoln, Gandhi, and Ohsawa taught us supreme judgment which they learned from their mothers. Therefore, mother is the greatest spiritual educator. However, she can also be the educator of the lazy, the dishonest, and the troubled. Thus the future of the world – happiness or unhappiness, peace or war, health or sickness – depends on the mother.

She is the most influential educator.

Why Macrobiotics Recommends Grains

When I lectured on the macrobiotic diet to teachers, nurses, doctors, and medical students at the University of California at Berkeley's School of Nutrition, one of the questions was why macrobiotics recommends so much grains (carbohydrates). (Actually, only two questions were asked; the other was, how does the macrobiotic diet supply enough vitamin B_{12}?)

I answered that, judging from their shapes, our thirty-two teeth consist of twenty for grains, eight for vegetables, and four for meats. Therefore, it is natural to eat foods in this proportion. Another reason I mentioned was the social and economic point of view. In other words, grain is the cheapest and most abundant source of calories, and only grains can prevent world hunger. However, I was not able to give sound nutritional or medical reasoning as to why we recommend grain. Not only was I unable to do this, but to my knowledge no macrobiotic person has ever explained why we should eat mostly grain – that is to say, 50 to 60 percent of the diet. Even Ohsawa didn't give an answer for this.

It was my big joy and surprise when the *U.S. Dietary Goals*, published by the Senate Select Committee on Nutrition in 1977, stated its first goal as follows: "Increase carbohydrate consumption to account for approximately 55 to 60 percent of the energy intake." The report explains the reason for this statement as follows.

First, a diet high in complex carbohydrates may reduce the risk of heart disease. "Most population groups with a low incidence of coronary heart disease consume from 65 to 85 percent of their total energy in the form of carbohydrates derived from whole grains and tubers." (*Present Knowledge in Nutrition*, by Drs. William E. and Sonja J. Connor, The Nutrition Foundation, 1976.) *Dietary Goals* continues:

> In their report, Drs. Connor conclude that high carbohydrate diets are quite appropriate for both normal individuals and for most of those with hyperlipidemia (high levels of fat in the blood), provided that the carbohydrate is largely derived from grains and tubers. The use of high (complex) carbohydrates by civilized man has an historical basis, is economically sound, and shows a clear indication of causing less rather than more disease, especially in the coronary heart disease-hyperlipidemia area. . . .
>
> The Connors also report that the high complex carbohydrate diet is important in the treatment of diabetes because it reduces the threat of atherosclerosis and hyperlipidemia, which are common to diabetics, by lowering cholesterol and saturated fat levels. The Connors note that some diabetics find a carbohydrate diet also results in improved glucose tolerances; in others, insulin requirements have been stabilized.

Another reason to increase carbohydrate intake is that it increases fiber consumption. "Dr. Denis P. Burkitt, among the first advocates of the high-fiber diet, has postulated that an increase in fiber consumption, preferably natural fiber rather than fiber added to refined products such as white bread, will markedly reduce the incidence of bowel cancer and other diseases, primarily those of the intestine." (*Dietary Goals.*)

Finally, an increase in the consumption of complex carbohydrates is likely to ease the problem of weight control. Professor Olaf Mickelson of Michigan State University reports in *General Foods World*, July 1985:

Contrary to what most people think, bread in large amounts is an ideal food in a weight-reducing regimen. Recent work in our laboratory indicates that slightly overweight young men lost weight in a painless and practically effortless manner when they included twelve slices of bread per day in their program. That bread was eaten with their meals. As a result, they became satiated before they consumed their usual quota of calories. The subjects were admonished to restrict those foods that were concentrated sources of energy; otherwise, they were free to eat as much as they desired. In eight weeks, the average weight loss for each subject was 12.7 pounds.

The U.S. Senate's recommendation of high carbohydrate consumption is based on statistics; however, it lacks scientific explanation. The best nutritional explanation of this is in *Live Longer Now*, Nathan Pritikin's bestseller. According to this book, the explanation is like this. In order to live, we need a certain amount of calories every day which are supplied by the consumption of protein, fat, and/or carbohydrate. Within this, we cannot depend too much on protein because it produces poisons. The next element eliminated at first was carbohydrate, because all carbohydrates are made of simple sugar, which will give a bad effect when eaten in quantity. Therefore, nutritionists formerly recommended high fats for the source of energy. Then, Ancel Keys's revolutionary theory came. He found during a fifteen-year study of 281 businessmen that high cholesterol and high blood pressure were the main differences between those who died of heart disease and those who did not. Keys later conducted a massive study involving more than twelve thousand people from seven different countries. Here, Dr. Keys found that fats in the blood also correlated with high incidence of heart disease as well as high cholesterol in the blood.

Then scientists studied primitive peoples such as the

Bantus, New Guineans, and Ecuadorians. The result was always the same. Low fat/low cholesterol meant a low incidence of heart disease. Furthermore, in order to prove that this was not the result of a natural immunity to heart disease in those people, Keys studied the Japanese population in three different environments, as reported in *Live Longer Now* (Keys, A., et al., Lessons From Serum Cholesterol Studies in Japan, Hawaii, and Los Angeles, Ann. Int. Med., 48:83-94, 1958). "It was found that the Japanese group in Japan had a very low incidence of heart disease. The Japanese group in Hawaii, on the other hand, had a significantly higher incidence of heart disease, while the Japanese group in Los Angeles evidenced a rate of heart disease equal to that suffered by Americans." By this study it is revealed that protection from heart disease among Japanese is not by natural immunity but from their diet.

During the twenty years between 1950 and 1970, many laboratory experiments were conducted to find out if diet could cause heart disease in animals. In 1959 a diet very much like what many Americans eat every day – about 42 percent fat and about one-fiftieth of an ounce of cholesterol per day – was found to produce heart trouble in monkeys. Since that time the experiment has been repeated many times on different animals by many researchers. The results were always identical – that is, high fat and high cholesterol produce heart disease. At one time, unsaturated fats were considered beneficial to heart disease, but experiments showed that they were no better than saturated fats (Friedman, M., et. al., JAMA 193:882, 1965; Bierenbaum, M., et.al., Circulation 42:943, 1970).

Thus the study of heart disease eliminated the high-fat diet. The only way left to supply enough energy is with a high-carbohydrate diet. However, a diet high in carbohydrates has been avoided by diabetics due to the belief that consumption of carbohydrates might cause a patient to pass into a diabetic coma, a condition suffered when they consume sugar. Ironically, the high carbohydrate diet is recommendable not only to heart disease patients but to diabetics as well. I.M. Rabinowitch in 1935, Wolf and Priess in 1956, and W.E. Connor in 1963 studied a low-fat (high-carbohydrate) dietary treatment of diabetes. They all found that patients fared far better on low-fat diets than on other diabetes-control regimens (*Live Longer Now*, p. 55).

In reality, what scientists learned was that there is a vital difference between complex carbohydrates and simple carbohydrates. "Simple carbohydrates in the diet convert to fats; they increase blood fats and certain diabetic symptoms. On the other hand, complex carbohydrates have just the opposite effect." (*Live Longer Now*, p. 56.)

According to Pritikin, a diet of simple carbohydrates increases both fat and cholesterol. Thus what is not good for diabetes is also not good for heart disease. He writes (p. 59), "Experience with low-fat diets and evidence of the lack of diabetes in primitive groups of people who have essentially low-fat diets have brought forth the low-fat, high-carbohydrate diet as the only viable means for preventing and treating diabetes in most cases. The carbohydrates in such a diet must of necessity exclude the simple carbohydrates – table sugar, honey, molasses, and so forth . . ."

From the macrobiotic point of view, food is the foundation of life and life is a manifestation of food. Therefore, the mechanism of evolution can be explained from the standpoint of foods. About 4.5 billion years ago the earth was covered by water (inorganic elements), some of which was then converted (about 3.5 billion years ago) to carbohydrate, fat, or protein – that is to say, organic matter. About 3 billion years ago, bacteria appeared in the water; probably, lightning was the cause of this transmutation from organic matter to bacteria. These bacteria were the first living things (plant life) on the earth.

From these simple plants, photosynthetic plankton arose. Some of these vegetable plankton became more active (yang) due to the weather becoming colder (which is yin). In the cold weather, the yin vegetable world would die out and the yang would survive. Therefore, living organisms which fed on such yang plankton naturally became more yang. When vegetal plankton becomes yang, it transmutes to animal plankton; this happened about 1.5 billion years ago. About a billion years ago, sponges (animal life) and shellfish (500 million years ago) followed. It was about 400 million years ago that other fishes appeared. When the great land masses appeared, about 300 million years ago, some plants stayed there and became land plants. Some fish adapted to both ocean and land environments and became amphibians. About 250 million years ago, ferns and mosses were abundant; reptiles arose, followed by insects. At this time (about 200 million years ago) the climate was very warm and dinosaurs and giant ferns predominated. Next, as the climate began swinging back to the cold side again, ferns began dying out and were replaced by early gymnosperms (plants whose seeds are exposed) about 150 million years ago. Animals which can feed on these foods – birds and mammals – appeared. Then about 100 million years ago, angiosperms (plants whose seeds are enclosed in an ovary) arose, making a more yang food for animals. Some more yang animals preyed on others. Thus carnivorous mammals started. Others fled to the trees to escape. This was the origin, about 75 million years ago, of the fruitarian primates. Then, about 50 million years ago, owing mainly to the thinning out of the trees, many primates had to leave the trees. This was the origin of apes and monkeys. (These animals, although they continued to get their food from the trees, were able to live either on land or in the trees.)

The rise of herbs began about 25 million years ago. Fruitarian apes found grains and began eating them. They began standing up about 10 million years ago. In my opinion, eating grains made the apes stand up, and caused the development of their brains. As a result of standing up, their hands were freed from the function of supporting the body and manual dexterity developed. This was the origin, about 5 million years ago, of homo faber – the tool maker. Then about 1 million years ago they discovered fire, and this is the origin of homo sapiens – man.

It took hundreds of thousands of years from the appearance of the first man to develop the man of agriculture. The *Encyclopedia Britannica* states, "For hundreds of thousands of years, during the Paleolithic Period, or Old Stone Age, primitive men lived on natural resources, both animal and vegetable. Paleolithic man was differentiated from other animals by little more than the fact that his lesser physical strength and natural weapons were compensated for by the tools and weapons that his greater mental development enabled him to provide." In my opinion, this was the result of his eating grains. The *Britannica* continues:

> The recession of the ice cap at the end of the last glaciation brought a different climate to the region at approximately 10,000 B.C. The challenge of this change in environment resulted in an enormous step forward, in that man began to seek to control his environment – that is, he began to cultivate plants and domesticate animals. Having taken this step, he was no longer forced to follow the seasonal migration of animals or growth of grains but could produce his own food supply within reach of his home. Settlement is dependent on a food supply controlled by means of agriculture and stock herding, and from the first village settlements developed the first town and, ultimately, civilization.

Babylonia, Egypt, Greece, and Rome were all based on the growing of wheat, barley, and millet. The ancient cultures of India, China, and Japan were based on the rice crop. The pre-Columbian people of the Inca, Maya, and Aztec civilizations in the New World depended on Indian corn (maize) for their daily bread. Therefore, some civilizations created myths which consider grain as their life-giving god or goddess, and some created codes of foods based on grains. The Mormon religion states, "All grain is ordained for the use of man and of beasts, to be staff of life, not only for man but for the beasts of the field, and the fowls of heaven, and all wild animals that run or creep on the earth." (Chapter 25, *A Marvelous Work and a Wonder*, LeGrand Richards, Deseret Book Co., 1969.)

According to the Gegu Ceremony Book (written in 804 A.D.), the twenty-first emperor of Japan, Emperor Yuryaku, constructed the Ise Shrine (in 457 A.D.) which enshrined the goddess Amaterasu, the highest goddess of the Japanese Shinto religion. One night, Emperor Yuryaku dreamed an appearance of Goddess Amaterasu who told him, "I am appreciative of you enshrining me, but you made a bad mistake neglecting Toyouke No Okami, the Rice God, whom I admire most. Please bring him here soon." Surprised, Emperor Yuryaku started constructing a shrine for Toyouke No Okami the next day. This shrine is called Gegu (guest shrine) and the shrine for Amaterasu is called Naigu (the domestic shrine). Japanese mythology also tells that Amaterasu Ohmikami made a declaration saying the people of Japan should eat rice as their main food. This goddess's declaration was one of the most important commandments of Japan. However, this has been forgotten except by a few such as George Ohsawa.

In conclusion, macrobiotics recommends grains as a main food (50 to 60 percent of foods normally eaten) for the following reasons:

1. Man evolved from unicellular organisms to present homo sapiens through a change of foods. At the present stage, man's principal food is grains because the proportion of our

dentition indicates: ⅝ grains; ¼ vegetables; and ⅛ animal foods.

2. The potassium/sodium ratio of grain is very close to that of the body cells – 10 to 1 – so it is an ideal basic material for body maintenance and building.

3. Carbohydrates contained in whole grains are complex carbohydrates, which change to glucose very slowly. Therefore, eating grains does not upset our sugar metabolism.

4. A high protein diet (exceeding about 16 percent of caloric intake) causes a negative mineral balance, mainly calcium loss, and therefore acidifies the body fluid. Thus, protein cannot be our main food. According to recent research, fats (either saturated or unsaturated) cause atherosclerosis, and therefore heart disease and diabetes. Thus fat, even though it is the highest energy source within human foods, cannot be a main food. Complex carbohydrates should be the main source of our calories.

5. Nutritionally speaking, whole grains – one-seeded fruits – contain mainly carbohydrates, some fats, some proteins, and minerals and vitamins. Many nutritionists recommend complex carbohydrates as the best food for man.

6. Economically speaking, grains are the cheapest source of calories and other nutrients. Grains are also compact and dry, so they store well without spoiling.

7. Grains are the most abundantly grown foods in the world. Only grain can sustain the entire population of the world, if eaten in a whole (unrefined) form. Grain is the highest calorie producer from a given area of land compared with other foods. Approximately twenty to thirty people can live from one acre of land if they consume their nutrients from grains; by contrast, one cow needs ten to fifteen acres for a year of grazing and will yield 300 or 400 pounds of meat. Since the average individual who is a meat eater consumes at least 250 pounds per year (a conservative estimate), it is quite apparent

that the use of meat as a principal food does not make good sense. It fosters land shortage, as there is just not enough land to feed a world of carnivores. What is bound to result, as history proves, is conflict. Many a war in the past has been fought over land, and the prospect for the future is not bright. War is inevitable due to the shortage of food in the future on this planet Earth unless we consume grains as the main food. (About 50 percent of our foods consumed should be grains and legumes.)

The Chinese character wa (和) translates in English to 'peace' or 'harmony'. This is a combination of two letters; 禾 is cereal plants, and 口 is mouth. Therefore, this character suggests that eating grains is peace. There are many peace movements nowadays. However, one who does not live on whole grains may lead such a movement by mere sentimental action.

8. Grains – particularly wheat, rice, and corn – have been used down through the centuries as the basis for diet. Their value for nutrition and taste has been tested and proven by millions of people over thousands of years of time.

9. According to Oriental philosophy (or the order of the universe), yang depends on yin (and, yang attracts yin). Therefore, yang animals (man included) should depend on the plant world for sustenance. Among plants, grains are the most yang (compact, dry, rich in sodium, etc.) and are the best food for man in the vegetable kingdom for maintaining a yang condition. This is a very good reason grain is recommended for man.

10. Lastly, we know by our experience and that of thousands of others that grains as a main food satisfy our hunger and our taste. They are a great, tasty food. Not only that, but they improve our health without exception if eaten unrefined, cooked properly, and consumed moderately.

For these reasons we recommend grains as our main food.

August 1982

U.S. Economics

In April of 1982, I was told that the AM International Corporation (Addressograph Multigraph Corporation), one of the major office machine companies in the United States for fifty-nine years, had just declared bankruptcy. Two years ago we bought a typesetting machine made by them and are still paying its cost. Their bankruptcy surprised many business people. The reason for bankruptcy was too much debt ($465 million in 1982), with business declining. The loss was $245 million in 1981.

A month after AM declared bankruptcy, Braniff Airlines did the same. Their reason was too-high interest rates, making loans too expensive for the purchase of new airplanes.

The big farm equipment company, International Harvester, lost $393 million in 1981 and was estimated to lose $518 million in 1982. They are asking help in financing from some Japanese companies. Sales fell drastically because American farmers are postponing farm equipment purchase due to the high interest rates.

Even RCA, one of the biggest names in electronic and appliance manufacture, is in bad shape with a debt of $3 billion. It is trying to sell its subsidiary, Hertz Rent-A-Car, to a tire company for $700 million in order to reduce the debt. And A&P, once the largest supermarket chain in the country, is reducing its number of stores from 3600 to 1200.

The Oakland-based Fidelity Savings and Loan Association was rumored of bankruptcy, so customers lined up for withdrawal. From eighty branches in Oakland, $25 million was withdrawn in one day. Finally, the federal government and the Savings & Loan Insurance Company took over to avoid the bankruptcy.

Dun & Bradstreet reported 17,043 business bankruptcies last year which is next only to 1961 when bankruptcies amounted to 17,075. This year is even worse. There were 3065 bankruptcies in the first seven weeks, 50 percent more than a year earlier.

The ill symptoms of U.S. economics are not only bankruptcy but also slow business, especially in the housing and auto manufacturing industries. The general manager of General Motors said, "If the economy does not turn by the end of this year, it will be the beginning of the end for the U.S. auto industry." (*Time*, March 8, 1982.)

Making the American economy worse is its increasing unemployment. *Time*, May 17, 1982 reports, "Joblessness has replaced inflation as the no. 1 concern of Americans. According to a Gallup poll taken last month, 44 percent of the public believe that unemployment is the most important problem facing the U.S." Unemployment now is a very serious problem, reaching a record high of 9.4 percent in May. On June 15th, a Wisconsin paper reported that Michigan, Ohio, Wisconsin, and Indiana each reached over 14 percent unemployment as well as Alabama and Washington. Even California had over 9.7 percent unemployment.

In Michigan and Ohio, efforts to attract new industry and retain workers are drying up for lack of money. This is caused mainly by high interest rates.

As mentioned previously, one of the main causes of the bankruptcies is the high interest rate, and the same is applied to the high rate of unemployment.

Why are interest rates so high? Everywhere President Reagan goes, people ask him the same question. He was even asked this by eighth-grade students at St. Peter's School in Geneva, Illinois. Those students were confused by his answer, according to *Time*, May 3, 1982. It seems to me it is not only those young students who are confused by Reagan's explanation but almost anyone – from those who operate their own businesses to the family owner who wants to buy his own house. When interest rates are high, businessmen can't borrow money from banks, and family men can't buy a home. Then, businesses may fold, no houses are sold, and new cars don't move. The result is many bankruptcies, slow business in lumber and automobiles, and much more.

The interest rates are the price for borrowing money and are determined by the balance between the supply and the demand for money. If not enough money circulates, the interest rate goes up. The controller of the amount of money is the Federal Reserve Board. Since the Reserve Board doesn't want inflation, it makes less money. This is the reason the interest rate goes up.

Therefore, the only way to lower the interest rate is to reduce the demand for money. In the U.S., the biggest money demand is made by the federal government. The government borrows from the Federal Reserve Bank to balance out their budget deficit which will be about $100 billion in 1983 (10 percent of the total tax).

Since the government demands so much money, available funds to business or individuals goes down. Therefore the interest rate goes up. Why does the government demand so much money? Because its military budget is too big to be covered by federal taxes. (The government's budget for military spending in 1983 is $215 billion.)

The easiest way to solve the economic situation in this country would be to cut military spending by $100 billion so that the government has no need to borrow money from the Federal Reserve Board. This is the first step for economic recovery in this country. Japan is a good example of this. After surrendering to allied forces at the end of World War II, Japan was forced to change her constitution such that she would have no military forces except a small defending force. Since then she has been enjoying a low military budget and therefore low taxes. One of the main reasons Japan made so fast an economic recovery after the war is her low taxes. With low taxes, the Japanese could save and invest more of their income than Americans. Now the American government is asking Japan to spend more money for military forces and weapons. Ironically, this is against the Japanese Constitution which she was obliged to form by the United States.

It is dangerous and useless to spend so much money on military weapons. Today's weapons, especially nuclear weapons, are so powerful that we don't need many. One hydrogen bomb will be more destructive than more than a hundred thousand of the atomic bombs which destroyed Hiroshima and Nagasaki and killed 350,000 people thirty-seven years ago.

Nichidatsu Fujii, a famous Japanese monk who led a peace march from Japan to the United States, wrote in *The Time Has Come* that both the United States and the Soviet Union now possess stockpiles of nuclear warheads equivalent to one million times those used on Hiroshima and Nagasaki. Therefore, 350 billion people would be killed by these nuclear weapons in case of an outbreak of total nuclear warfare. This means that fifty times the world population would be killed in a second were the U.S.A. and the Soviet Union to start a nuclear war. It took six years to kill approximately 50 million soldiers and innocents during World War II. It will only require a second in total nuclear warfare to kill fifty times the total world population.

It is my understanding that the United States and the Soviet

Union have mutually agreed to preserve their lands as a sanctuary where strategic nuclear weapons are not to be used. They schemed to have nuclear warfare only in the territories of other smaller and weaker nations or satellite countries.

However, it is not only the United States and the Soviet Union who possess nuclear powers; according to the International Atomic Energy Agency, there are some 340 research reactors and 475 power reactors in operation or under construction in a total of forty-six nations (*Time*, June 22, 1981). In fact, it seems that any country could produce a nuclear bomb if they really wanted.

Making the situation worse is the fact that nuclear know-how might eventually pass to international terrorists as feared by Princeton physicist Theodore Taylor, a one-time atom bomb designer. Nobody can deny that, sometime, a terrorist or another Hinckley may explode a homemade A-bomb and trigger a chain reaction leading to World War III.

A fear that Europeans could be incinerated in a war between the superpowers (U.S. and Russia) was the driving force of the 1981 peace march in Bonn. About seven months later, on June 12, 1982, nearly half a million people from all over the world protested against nuclear weapons at an armaments gathering in New York's Central Park. The demonstration was the largest gathering in New York City in one day and one place, and was well-planned and peaceful. There was not the feeling of fear from demonstrators as had been present at the Bonn demonstration. People's consciousness is apparently improving. However, I had a thought similar to that expressed by New York mayor Edward Koch: "It is terrific to try to affect the conscience of the world. It is just regrettable they don't have a similar demonstration in Moscow." (*Time*, June 21, 1982.)

Spending $134 billion and $118 billion respectively in 1981, the U.S.A. and Russia were the most armed countries in the world. Therefore, it is most important for the world politically as well as economically that these two countries reach an agreement to stop further armament.

It is ideal that all countries in the world give up arms and soldiers. Is it a daydream to think of such a world? Is it a utopian and childish idea to think of such a world? I used to think so, but I think differently now.

We should ask why we have soldiers and armaments. We should study the way to eliminate them as Japan did following her surrender to the allied forces. Without such study, just sentimental disarmament demonstrations will not stop a World War III which may be starting already.

In my opinion, one of the reasons many governments prepare (nuclear) weapons is the fear of an energy shortage. Our life depends heavily on oil or petro-products. Every country depends on imported oil, excepting a few. Acquiring oil is the main purpose of having military weapons. Therefore, in order to avoid acquiring so many weapons, we have to overcome the oil dependency.

There are two ways to do this. One is to learn to use fewer petro-products such as plastic bags, synthetic clothing, etc. Another is to develop alternative energy such as solar, wind, ocean wave, etc. Infinite energy exists in the whole universe. We have to find an atomic energy without yin radiation. We have to investigate all sources of energy. What is the source of the energy which creates the rotation of the earth, its own rotation as well as its movement around the sun? How is the sun's energy created? There are many energies in ourselves. How does the heart beat? What mechanism makes the heart beat from before birth until death without a second's rest? What makes the ocean waves which have such tremendous energy?

Only when we find or utilize alternative sources of energy which are quantitatively and economically available to the world population of six billion will the present world crisis be overcome. All governments should spend money for researching alternative energy sources instead of spending for weapons and war preparations.

Another reason to prepare arms is the fear of hunger. In today's political world, food is a weapon. Governments prepare weapons in order to secure foods. This is only true for countries where people depend on animal foods. The reason for this is that there is not enough grazing land in the world to produce enough animal foods (excepting fish) to supply the calorie and protein quota of the world population. One cow requires about ten acres of land and supplies 450 pounds of meat which will support only one person a year. On the other hand, if we cultivate grains, one acre produces about 5000 pounds of grains which can support about twenty persons a year calorie-wise. Therefore, if we were to depend on grains as a main food, there would be no shortage of land to produce enough food on the earth. Dependence on animal food creates a shortage of land and consequently food. Therefore, countries must fight each other in order to increase their land. For this, preparations for war and stockpiling of weapons are inevitable.

In order to achieve a sound economy, we must teach that grains are the best basic food.

Clearly, the economic situation in the U.S.A. is not bright. As long as the government spends lots of money on weaponries, we will be taxed highly and interest rates and the inflation rate will continue to be high. Furthermore, scarcity of foods, epidemics of diseases, and high crime rates may threaten our life. In such a doomsday, the important thing is that we keep ourselves healthy in body as well as mind. For the healthy body, I recommend a macrobiotic diet – high grain, vegetables, whole foods, and no chemicals. This is a sane, economical, and peace-bringing diet. The leaders of all nations should observe this diet. If ten thousand government officials around the world were to observe this diet, wars between nations would cease to exist. The reason for this is that a macrobiotic diet will eliminate attitudes of aggressive mentality and fear, so that much of the cause of war would be dissolved.

However, it is difficult to expect ten thousand world leaders to observe a macrobiotic diet. Therefore, world peace cannot be expected soon. Doomsday will continue. Nuclear war may happen. One who survives this war is one who knows health principles and can practice them in daily life. The macrobiotic diet proved its healing and survival power during atomic war at the St. Francis Hospital in Nagasaki. One should start the diet as soon as possible, not only for heart attacks but also for the possibility of nuclear attack.

For a healthy mind, I recommend living with the principle of Lao Tsu, which is moderation. The fall of Braniff Airways resulted from an overly ambitious expansion program in the late 1970s. They did not manage the company with moderation. This is the case with many other bankruptcies.

Not only businesses but governments should operate with the principle of moderation. Since the American government spends without moderation, America's national debt reached over $1 trillion, interest alone over $100 billion, in June of 1982. This is one of the reasons the interest rate in America is so high, as mentioned earlier.

Moderation is not only for businesses and governments but also for individuals and families. In other words, we have to practice moderation in the food we eat, clothes we wear, and houses we live in.

According to *Time* (May 31, 1982), millions of Americans are in trouble because the personal debt in 1981 averaged out to $6,737 for every citizen. And more and more often, people cannot pay; personal bankruptcies reached 179,194 in 1978, and 456,914 in 1981. The same magazine reports on a lawyer and his wife who together earned $40,000 a year. They have a new car and new kitchen. They look like the All-American Family living the All-American Dream. They are also broke. They are not only broke, but $18,000 in debt. Why did this happen? Because they forgot the principle of moderation, once taught by Benjamin Franklin. Today's principle of living is to stretch money out as much as possible – spend now, pay later; borrow first, worry later.

When people lose moderation – another name for balance or harmony – they are inviting trouble. *Time* continues:

> They went into debt because cheap credit made living easy and because inflation seemed to guarantee big annual salary increases and the prospect of repaying debts with cheaper dollars. But now many consumers face very unpleasant consequences. The recession and high interest rates threaten all its illusions. . . . "For people to admit they can't afford the things they want means they are placing themselves in a position of weakness," says Edward J. Khantzian, associate professor of psychiatry at Harvard Medical School. "They have to say no to themselves, and nobody likes to do that. It all boils down to the inability to accept limit."

This means Americans lost the principle of moderation and balance. Not only individuals, but government officials and lawmakers – all lost moderation. This is the cause of the present-day economic trouble in America. As long as there are no balanced budgets in the government, the American economy will continue to worsen until a final disaster which may be World War III in fifteen years, unless we can change this trend.

In conclusion, in these economically uncertain days, true wealth will not be measured by money in banks or insurance policies. True wealth will be measured by having plenty of grains, a good source of water nearby, good health, a small but well-mulched garden, a safe and warm house which is not too big, and a number of good family members and friends.

The Essence of Macrobiotics
Lecture at French Meadows Summer Camp

Today I am speaking of very, very basic macrobiotics.

You have to understand the essence of macrobiotics. Curing cancer, tuberculosis, or heart disease is not the essence – that is just the result, the end product or byproduct. You have to understand the main thing, the essence, of macrobiotics; then the byproduct comes naturally. If you do it the other way, it is very difficult. If you want to try and cure disease first, it is very difficult; but if you follow the mainstream essence, then the rest comes naturally. What is the macrobiotic essence?

Always when you are thinking, you think in two terms – of course, yin and yang. There is the yin side of macrobiotics and there is the yang side. The yin side of macrobiotics is spirit – you cannot see, touch, feel, or eat it. The yang side of macrobiotics has substance – we call it diet, or physicality, or physiology. You can see it, touch it, feel it. Most people start on the yang side of macrobiotics and many stay on the yang side only, never reaching the yin side. I started on the yin side and much later started the yang side. That is okay. Many start on the yang side and reach the yin side much later. That is okay too. But in the end, you have to have both. It is up to you which side you want to start with.

Let's talk about the yang side first, then the yin side. The yang side includes diet and is familiar to you. The essence of the macrobiotic diet is grain. You can forget about the

172

vegetables, seaweeds, condiments, etc. – the main food is grain. That is why Ohsawa recommended the number seven diet. But in order to live on just grain you have to be healthy; therefore, I recommend the grain diet only to advanced macrobiotic students. What do vegetables do in our body? They give us enzymes and co-enzymes, and small amounts of carbohydrates, protein, and fats – very little. These three sustain our life and build blood and cells, and are supplied mainly by grains. We depend on vegetables and sea vegetables for enzymes and co-enzymes. What are enzymes? They are a promoter, speeding up chemical reactions. If we don't have enzymes, our chemical reactions are very slow and don't meet the requirements for breaking up and assimilating our food. Sometimes enzymes are not enough for this action, and help is needed. The helpers are called co-enzymes; another name for them is vitamins. Vitamins are produced only in vegetables. So if you don't have enough enzymes you have to eat vegetables – that is why we eat vegetables.

When you become very healthy, it seems you don't need vegetables as much. Some mountain men in Japan live just on seeds and nuts – they have enough enzymes and vitamins. We have not reached such a condition yet, so we have to have some vegetables, especially at the beginning. If you have been eating lots of animal foods, as you probably have been, then you lack many enzymes and co-enzymes. Therefore, when you came to macrobiotics you needed lots of vegetables and seaweeds, etc., at the start. As you improve your health, gradually you don't need as many vegetables. But in the beginning you needed lots. So, the essence of the diet changes as your health changes.

As your condition changes, your requirements change. Make no mistake, dietary needs are not the same for everybody; and even for the same person it is not the same every day, all the time. You have to understand the essence of essence: Change. There is no clear-cut sentence, This is it; there is no such thing in macrobiotics. As your condition improves, things change. Sometimes you need much vegetables, seaweeds, sesame salt, or this or that – but sometimes not so much. So please remember, what you need is changing, always changing. Many mistakes are often made. For example, parents cannot take salt, so they don't give any to their children, and the children become sick. What happened? The parents took animal foods for many long years and have an accumulation of salt. Therefore, salt is not so essential or necessary for them. But if their babies have been grown macrobiotically, it is essential for them to be taking salt in some form. So the essential needs of parents and their children are different in such cases. This must be understood. And things are different from person to person.

While our ancestors, probably from any race or culture, knew thousands of years ago that man's main food is grain, modern science recognized this fact only very recently. Many countries have religions telling that grain is the main food. In Roman religion, Ceres was worshipped as the goddess of food plants. In Mexico and for the Native Americans, corn is worshipped as the main food. In Japan, there is the goddess of rice. Rice was considered the most important food two thousand years ago; the rice goddess told the Japanese, "If you eat rice," of course whole grain rice, "the Japanese race will never die out." But almost two thousand years after Christ, in about 1976, science and the American government finally recognized grain as the main food.

Our main source of energy comes from three types of nutrients: carbohydrates, protein, and fats. Modern nutritional science had been searching for the most important one. Carbohydrates were not chosen because they are mainly made of complex sugars, and sugar has caused a lot of trouble, primarily diabetes. So carbohydrates were eliminated. Next we eliminated fats as a primary nutrition source; around 1960

Ancel Keys found that our biggest health enemy – arteriosclerosis, or heart disease – was caused by too much fat in our diet. The remainder is protein, but protein was soon found not such a good main energy source due to its tendency to remove minerals and acidify the body. So in this century, we found that no food was good – neither carbohydrates, protein, nor fats. Then, one scientist experimented with whole grains, giving them to diabetics. It was considered very dangerous to give sugar to diabetics, but this doctor gave them whole grains and they were cured. So scientists finally recognized that sugar and whole grains are different. This is science. They didn't realize until so recently that sugar and whole grains are different. We had been telling them. I don't know how he found it but Ohsawa said many years ago to give whole grains to diabetics, and they didn't listen. Almost eighty years ago, the original macrobiotic doctor in Japan, Sagen Ishizuka, said the same thing, and it was also known two thousand years ago. Whole grains – complex carbohydrates – are made of sugar, so scientists thought grain was the same as simple sugars. When they realized the difference, then grains were considered more important.

The British scientist Denis Burkitt worked at an African hospital and realized the natives had no heart disease. In his five years at the hospital no natives came with heart disease, only whites and some natives who were living in the city. He was very curious – what was the difference? His conclusion was diet: whole grains.

These findings, along with the U.S. Senate recommendation that unrefined grains should comprise 55 percent of our diet, brought grains into greater prominence.

Finally, of dietetic essence: Please chew well. As you know, grains are mainly carbohydrates, which are digested mostly by saliva. If they are not well mixed with saliva, they are difficult to digest. So chew very well.

This is the essence of the yang side of macrobiotics.

Now for the yin side of macrobiotics – the spiritual side. I more emphasize the spiritual side than the physical side of macrobiotics. To understand the spiritual side of macrobiotics, first of all you have to understand what life is. What is life? Actually, to understand this would be graduation from macrobiotics. But you can do this. You are living. "You are living" means you know life. How many years have you been living – thirty years? You have been practicing your concept of life for thirty years. You know what life is – that is why you live. Consciousness doesn't know, but unconsciousness knows.

Life is not manifested without food. There is an invisible life which consumes definite food which is material and has life force, and gradually that invisible life materialized into something we can see. This 'great life' becomes manifested in the individual, and we have to understand that this individual life is naturally created healthy. If it is sick, that is not natural – something is wrong. So curing sickness is changing an unnatural thing back to natural. There is no need for any million-dollar gadget to cure sickness. Doctors are proud of the million-dollar scanning machine, but to me this is not so natural. To be healthy is natural; sickness is unnatural. So it is very easy to cure sickness, while it is very difficult to be sick. You have to understand this very clearly, it is the essence of macrobiotics; naturally you were not sick. People become sick and are often afraid: "Oh, I am going to die. I have to see the doctor and go to the hospital." Such mentality is because they don't clearly understand that sickness is not natural. Most of the time we are healthy, natural; sometimes, usually for short times in proportion to our lifespan, we are sick, unnatural. As soon as we become unnatural for a short time we are surprised, afraid, and sure that our sickness will continue forever. That makes us more sick, more than the original sickness. If you have a stomach pain, very soon the pain goes away because we have a natural life force which overcomes sickness and allows our health to manifest itself in its natural state. But when we have pain we take painkillers, etc., and that makes things even more unnatural. Then, the sickness goes deeper and deeper and deeper. That is what we are seeing now. Instead of allowing our life force to manifest, we manipulate and make things more unnatural. This is the essence: We have to understand that the natural life force is health. When you have such faith then you are very secure, your life is secure.

You also have to understand that when you are sick, the cause of the sickness is your mistake. It is not somebody or something else; it is you yourself, except in the case of a baby or child. After you start living on your own, all your sickness and unhappiness is caused by you – there is nothing to blame on anyone else. This was told by the Roman scholar Epictetus, and is essentially macrobiotic. Epictetus was a slave of the Roman Empire until the age of eighty – he was chained until he was eighty. But as a slave, he studied all the time. So one day the Roman emperor unchained him and made him his teacher. Epictetus then wrote four books; three volumes were lost and one remains, and in that book it is written, "Everyone is happy; if not, it is his own fault." He was a slave for eighty years. If you were sick for eighty years and were cured and could still say "Mea culpa," my fault – that is what he did.

I had a woman student two years ago with breast cancer – one side had been operated on and three months later the other side became malignant. She came to me, she wanted no further operations, and she studied the diet. She went home and started the diet, and three months later she came back to Vega Institute and studied more. When she came to stay at Vega she was in constant back pain, always taking painkillers. After one week, her pain was gone and there was no need for the pills. She was so happy. She said, "I am so happy I would like to live my life once more, exactly the same way." That means once more she would have cancer! Even if you have cancer you can be happy. That is amazing. That depends on your consciousness. Your sickness is physical, but happiness or unhappiness is your consciousness. This is very important. When you are sick, how can you be happy? If you eat very good food, in good proportions and good amounts, you can be happy even if you are sick. It is amazing. Your sickness cannot be cured overnight, but if you supply good food you can be happy. This is a very great relief. So please understand that our sickness and our unhappiness depend on ourselves.

If you understand that your sickness and your unhappiness totally depend on you, next comes the most difficult thing: There is nothing to complain about. You have to make a commitment, "I will not complain." This is an important essence of macrobiotics; when you complain, you are not macrobiotic. I will say that most difficulties in life begin with complaining.

I met a young couple on my lecture trip, they were almost separated. The husband had found a nice young girl, very pretty, and they were often meeting. The more his wife complained, the more the husband went to the beautiful girl – who didn't complain (yet!). Then he asked his wife, "Can I live two nights a week with her?" What can you say? So the wife said okay. She said okay, but inside she was not so happy, of course. But, understanding macrobiotics, she tried to embrace all. So the wife embraced that girlfriend – tried to – said okay. They asked me what I thought. I said, "Don't embrace. You can't embrace it. You can embrace spiritually but not physically. You cannot embrace two girls physically." He was not happy: "Tonight I am going to that beautiful girl and stay overnight." I said no. "If you are very highly spiritual, you cannot do that," I told him. They had confused the physical and the spiritual. The next morning his wife told me, "I made a big mistake. This trouble happened because I complained too much. I was always complaining to my husband; that's why he went to this other girl." She said to her husband, "I am sorry I complained so much." So they both understood. Some months later I met the husband again; he said things were okay, that he had separated from the young girlfriend. So, it is very important not to complain; if you complain, everything will break up.

This is very difficult in macrobiotics. Often, yang persons complain especially. Yin persons complain but don't show it. You have to talk instead of complaining. Complaining is destructive, but advice or suggestions or efforts to understand – these are important. If you have self-reflected and want to say something to her, then it is not complaining; but if your ego says, "I don't want this, this, this," then you are complaining. There is a very delicate difference between these two. If you are really sincere in your thinking towards others, then it is not complaining. You just mask out your emotion.

So consider more before you complain. Just as you start to complain – swallow it. Almost as it starts coming out from your mouth, you swallow it – and digest it. Chew well! Then you will find it is not so important to complain. This attitude needs yin. Yang doesn't swallow – it all comes out right away with a yang person. With a yin person, a complaint goes back in again; sometimes it stays inside and is not digested and it causes 'constipation'. That is not good either, so we have to bring it back and digest it completely.

If you have something to complain about, you have to give a solution – how we can solve this problem – before complaining. If you think somebody made a mistake, give a suggestion instead of complaining. This may cause change – cause someone's behavior to change. In most cases, we cannot do this. If you can change someone's behavior, you are a very, very great man. If you cannot change someone's behavior, don't complain, because it is no use. The reason you are complaining is that you would like to change someone's behavior. If that doesn't work, there is no use to complain. Do you understand? Complaining is only worthwhile when that complaint is for mutual benefit, mutual happiness. If your complaining doesn't bring mutual happiness, it is not so good. If you want somebody's behavior to change, make suggestions. If you are a very great person, your suggestion will be accepted. If you are at the same level, the same emotional level, your suggestion is usually not accepted. This we have to think about.

You have to improve your spiritual power. To have your suggestions accepted, say "Please change your behavior" or "Your such-and-such actions make me sick; please change." Instead, you complain. Your suggestions can be accepted when you are very high spiritually. How can we make our spiritual powers high? That's our purpose. The purpose of macrobiotics is to make our spiritual power high, nothing else. To do so, we stop sugar. This is making our spiritual power high. Why? Because we like sugar. When we stop eating sugar, we elevate our spiritual power. When you stop eating meat you elevate your spiritual power because what you like is sensorial. Following what you like is sensorial judgment – sentimental, ego judgment – very low judgment. When you overcome this and you can control this sentimental sensorial judgment, you are of a higher level of spirit.

When beginning macrobiotics you stop what you have been liking. If you liked cheese, you stopped cheese. So you improve your spiritual power very much at the beginning. At first you don't much like rice, but soon grains become very delicious after you stop sugar. Soon you like brown rice; that becomes your sensorial judgment. Next time, you stop brown rice – then you improve your sensorial judgment! Also, you quit something – smoking, for example. I tried to improve my judgment. I very much liked smoking for twenty-five years; it was very, very difficult to cut smoking, so I cut it. Then I cut fishing. I very much liked fishing, I was always thinking of fishing. What you like, cut. Stop. Then you are above sensorial/sentimental judgment. You like your husband, cut out husband. Very big problem!

Mostly you cannot do this. So do you understand the idea of sacrifice? Primitive people gave sacrifices to God. What you like the most, give to God. That means you will improve your sensorial/sentimental judgment. You have to give sacrifices. In Japanese tradition, for example, every day when you cook rice the first batch of rice is put in a bowl and given to God as a sacrifice. When you cook rice, you give the first batch to your neighbor so you eat less; that is sacrifice. If you practice that, you improve your spiritual life. Always live in sacrifice and you will improve. If you have a fruit tree, don't eat all the fruit yourself; give most of it to the neighbors. Giving is sacrifice. That is the spirit of macrobiotics. Give your time, that is a sacrifice – not only food. Give your time and help others. Time is money, time is life, so give your time. If you spend all your life only for yourself, that is not macrobiotic. If you live fifty years, give twenty-five years to others. That way you improve your judgment. Then people will start listening to you. If you don't improve yourself, other people don't listen. If you eat sugar and meat, as much as you want, nobody listens. Gandhi was a spiritual leader – 400 million Indians followed him because he himself had a high spirit. He controlled his eating and he had a strong power. That is what you will get – very, very strong power if you stay with macrobiotics.

If we have very strong spiritual power we can stop making so many nuclear bombs. First we have to be able to completely control ourselves. We have a strong power called supreme judgment, but we have been controlled by low judgment, sensorial and sentimental. If we have completely supreme judgment we can do anything.

Every day, every meal you are improving your spiritual

power. "I want to drink milk." You can stop it. "I want to eat ice cream." You can stop. Each time you overcome sensorial desire, you are improving. When you do eat by sensorial judgment, don't blame yourself; we are not perfect. But we know we are weak. Such reflection is important. Then, go back to macrobiotics.

These are my ideas on the essence of macrobiotics.

Thank you very much.

January 1983

The Tylenol Scare

The deaths of seven people caused by taking the painkiller drug Tylenol shocked everyone on October 6, 1982 and led the nation to great fear and uncertainty. This is a great terror because there are no clues for solving the mystery of why anyone would do such mass killing. Since then almost two months have passed. Neither criminals nor the cause have been found. According to *Newsweek* (October 11, 1982), the case happened like this: "The most likely theory was that someone had simply removed individual bottles from retail stores – selected, perhaps at random – filled a few capsules with the deadly poison, and sneaked them back onto the shelves for unsuspecting consumers to purchase. If so, the culprit could be virtually anyone – a disgruntled employee, for example, of McNeil or Johnson & Johnson or an overzealous competitor. But many experts thought that the culprit was simply a psychopath with a diabolical idea for anonymous murder."

If this is the work of the crazy, how can we avoid being victimized in the future? Perhaps all over-the-counter drugs will be sealed and tamper-proof. But there is no absolute guarantee that they will be safe, according to most authorities on future prevention of the possibility of drug tampering. In this confused and fearful incident, macrobiotic teaching and way of living can give light and relief. The following is my intention to reveal such a light.

183

Why did the Tylenol case happen? The drug-dependent mentality and habit is the real cause of the Tylenol case. *Time* magazine (October 11, 1982) reported:

> Adam Janus, 27, had a minor chest pain last Wednesday (October 6th) morning, so he went out and bought a bottle of Extra Strength Tylenol capsules. About an hour later in his home in the Chicago suburb of Arlington Heights, Janus suffered a cardiopulmonary collapse. He was rushed to Northwest Community Hospital, where doctors worked frantically to revive him. "Nothing seemed to help," said Dr. Thomas Kim, chief of the hospital's critical-care unit. "He suffered sudden death without warning. It was most unusual."

The rest of the six victims took Tylenol capsules and died in the same manner. People take non-prescription pills by habit. If someone has a headache, he buys a bottle of pills at a drugstore around the corner and takes one. Therefore, Americans spent about $1 billion a year for cold and cough drugs and $1.2 billion for internal analgesics in 1979. And the spending is going up every year (according to *Drug Topics, Marketing Guide*, Medical Economics Co., Oradell, New Jersey).

What an innocent and credulous mentality! People have been brainwashed to think that pain should be stopped at any cost and that if pain goes away, sickness is cured. This mentality – that which tries to stop pain at any cost, never thinking what is the real cause of the pain and what is the real cure – is the cause of the Tylenol case.

However, it seems to me nobody cares about such cause; instead they blame the way of packaging or the madness of society. For example, an article appeared in the *San Francisco Chronicle* (October 7, 1982) which said that politicians are calling for laws that would force companies to seal the mouth of every bottle of over-the-counter drugs. However, I feel that sealing bottles is not absolute protection against tampering.

The only absolute safety is in never getting such pain that you need to buy such drugs.

When I first heard of the Tylenol news, I thought this would be a benefactor to many people because they may stop taking over-the-counter drugs. I was wrong. The seven deaths by the cyanide-contaminated drug didn't change people's minds at all. One and a half months later, the *Chronicle* reported that "the seven deaths from cyanide in Extra Strength Tylenol Capsules have made the over-the-counter drug industry fearful that the public may shun its products. But apparently the public is less concerned about tampering than is the industry." The same paper reports that a consumer survey showed that 54 percent of them feel the non-prescription drugs are safe to take. Therefore, people will continue to buy pills believing they are their life-saver. However, the truth is that drugs are not safe even if they are not tampered with. Taking drugs is slow suicide, even if not lethal within fifteen minutes as in the Tylenol case.

Why is taking painkiller drugs slow suicide? The answer is very simple. Painkillers are a symptomatic remedy. It is not curing the sickness at all but just causing no feeling of pain. The worst thing is, painkillers not only stop pain but also stop the body's curing processes. For example, antihistamines or other kinds of drugs are given to stop a runny nose. People do not realize that this discharge is the body's natural curing system working by throwing out poisons.

In *Who Is Your Doctor and Why* (Alonzo J. Shadman, M.D., Keats Publishing, Inc., 1980), Dr. J. Haskel Kritzen is quoted from the *Journal of the Natural Medical Society:*

> However debilitating and annoying as the common cold is, it is nevertheless a beneficial effort of nature to relieve the body of accumulations of morbid waste. The cold is, therefore, a natural safety valve, a corrective measure to compensate for incomplete elimination. The

time, effort and money spent in the investigation of the common cold, the attempts to identify the specific germs, have thus far been fruitless. The only accomplished results are the manufacture of an unlimited variety of cold nostrums, serum and vaccines that are not only worthless, but are infinitely more harmful than the cold which they are intending to cure.

Doctors' prescriptions amounted to over $11 billion in 1979. Every American from the infant to the old spent at least $4 on drugs for colds, $4 for internal painkillers, and $50 for doctors' prescriptions per year. Why was so much money wasted? Drugs are not intended to cure but to worsen the condition. Once you take drugs, you need more. If drugs could cure at once, there would be no patients left and the drug manufacturers would be bankrupt. However, the truth is that the total drug consumption is increasing every year ($14 billion in 1975 and $20 billion in 1979).

Dr. Shadman, one of the rare medical doctors (surgeon) who opposed the use of drugs and believed in nature's healing power, writes how drug manufacturers deceive people:

> Each week every doctor's wastebasket is filled by an immense amount of literature extolling the virtues of an endless stream of drugs. Much of this literature is accompanied by samples of the drugs. I have been unable to find a single one of these products that has any *curative* action whatever, yet fourteen billion or more dollars are spent yearly for their purchase.
>
> The drug industry has one of the highest markups for its products of any industry in the nation. Its advertising budget is a sizeable percentage of the consumer price. Why spend so much for advertising? Because a market has to be created. You have to be made to believe that you must take such and such a pill at the first sign of a headache and such and such a pill at the first sign of stomach distress.

From a macrobiotic point of view, symptomatic medicine and analgesic drugs stop symptoms which are nature's toxin-elimination process. Therefore, the use of such drugs will create an accumulation of toxins inside the body. This leads to the malfunction of various organs, especially the kidneys, and finally to an acidic condition of the cellular fluids. In my opinion, this can lead to the formation of malignant cells. Therefore, the initiation of cancer cells can be caused by carcinogens and also the frequent use of symptomatic drugs. Each time one takes a painkiller or other symptomatic medicine, he is preparing cancer cell formation. Once cancer cells develop, the pain cannot be stopped by drugs.

The following is the therapeutic sequence of treatment given to Gabrielle, a nine-year-old girl, as taken from an article by Dr. Eugene Underhill, Jr. (reprinted in *Who Is Your Doctor and Why?*).

Bed rest and an aspirin every three hours.

Codeine prescribed by phone.

Possibility of Infectious Hepatitis or Catarrhal Jaundice.

More codeine but it didn't help.

Liver found to be enlarged.

Doctor thought patient seemed deranged but this was disproven.

Patient hospitalized in one of the best medical centers in the world.

Tests made but never dreamed there would be so many.

Took blood from arm twice, finger pricked several times.

Stuck with needle 17 times during first week, then lost count.

Finally decided it was Infectious Hepatitis.

Case was brought before weekly staff conference.

Doctors had many different opinions about what was wrong.

One doctor began to talk about an exploratory operation.

Mentioned possibility of a small tumor.

X-rays showed shadowy indentation in part of stomach.
Operation ordered.
Blood transfusion in preparation for operation.
Found tumor from spine invading everything.
Kind of tumor that does not respond to radiotherapy.
No drugs benefit this kind of cancer.
Tumor malignant and completely untreatable.
Patient in best possible hospital with best possible doctors.
Prescription filled for demerol.
Codeine injected, then another injection, then demerol.
More demerol, then phenobarbital.
Effect of demerol worn off, had to switch to morphine.
Flesh black and blue and very sore from so many injections.
Had frequent shots of vitamin K.
Shots of penicillin occasionally.
Gamma globulin twice because of measles in hospital.
Blood transfusion every few days, a long and exhausting procedure.
Symptoms shifted. Doctors could only guess at what was going on.
Even the patient observed the doctors don't know everything.
Luminol injection.
Paraldehyde for convulsions, repeated as necessary.
Note: *The patient died.*

This is only one of the sad stories of the sick whose only medicine is painkillers. This story shows that medicine has nothing to do with curing, but only stopping pain. However, the macrobiotic diet has proven to be far superior to any painkiller; even severe cancer patients have drastically reduced pain after following a strict version of the macrobiotic diet for a week or so.

In conclusion, the Tylenol case is a warning to people who are depending on drugs and doctors to alleviate pains and symptoms. It advises them to change their diet, so that no more drugs or painkillers are necessary.

We should have no headaches at all at any time. If you have, you have to stop taking sugar and sugary foods, soft drinks, and decrease total liquid intake. You may be surprised when simple dietary change cures the majority of headaches. Then you will wonder why we spend one billion dollars to stop such a simple pain.

January 1983

Happy New Year 1983

According to the Chinese calendar, this year is *Mizu-no-to I*: yin, Water, Boar. It is also the last year of the 60-year cycle. This is like a seed in the ground which is absorbing nutrients but is not yet germinated. This means that good things will not come out yet.

It seems to me that macrobiotics, at present, is in the ground and not known among the people. It is growing but not known. Dr. Sattilaro's articles, book, and TV appearances made quite a bit of publicity for macrobiotics, but the true value of macrobiotics has not been presented. Its potential, its validity, its eternalness are unknown to most.

I consulted the *I Ching* about the macrobiotic situation in 1983. It showed 54 (marriage) by 7 yang, 9 yang, 6 yin, 7 yang, 8 yin, 8 yin. This means macrobiotics causes the marriage of Eastern philosophy and Western medicine. However, there are many difficulties in this marriage because of the disorderliness in yin and yang. When I changed the second yang (9) to yin and the third yin (6) to yang, I got 49 (Change, or revolution).

The marriage between Eastern philosophy and Western medicine will cause a revolution in Western life and culture. Some of the germination for such a revolution will start later in this year. If such a revolution is realized, it will be the biggest revolution in human history.

190

February 1983

The Verdict

A magazine article on *The Verdict*, Paul Newman's movie, prompted me to see the movie when I was visiting Oakland during this past holiday season.

The story is about an alcoholic Irish Catholic lawyer who had four cases in three years and lost them all. Why? Nobody knew, but macrobiotics has an answer. Now he is bringing a malpractice suit against a doctor accused of misusing an anesthetic drug. He is so confident of winning that he refuses to accept the large amount of settlement money offered by the defense attorney.

However, his winning possibilities thin out one by one due to the defense attorney's cunning and shrewd protest and way of handling witnesses. His final and only hope of winning, the testimony of the nurse who actually administered the anesthetic to the patient by the doctor's order, was nullified by the defense attorney's shrewd argumentation.

He lost. He lost completely. Why? Common sense tells us that it was due to his alcoholism. Why can't he stop drinking? Because he is not happy. One way to become happy would be for him to change his lifestyle, including diet. This is not the story of the movie; however, the movie is very realistic. It does not give a simple happy ending. From beginning to end, the movie shows that the alcoholic lawyer must lose the case. The plots are set logically. From the macrobiotic viewpoint also,

191

he must fail because he is not living healthfully and therefore his judgment is not good. However, the poor lawyer's sincerity, which is the only virtue he had, caused a miracle. This miracle was brought by the jury system as practiced in the American trial by jury. What is the origin of the jury system? What are the pros and cons of the jury system? Such questions came to my mind.

The birth of the first idea of the jury system was in relatively ancient times, in old Greece. However, the jury system was abolished by the Greek emperor around 352 A.D. because it became too powerful and independent. Then, the jury system appeared in Scandinavia more than 1000 years ago. From Norway, the jury system went with the Normans to Iceland. However, the Scandinavians moved to Normandy (France) around 890 with the jury system. The system crossed the English channel again when William the Conqueror conquered the English in 1066 A.D.

When the English colonists arrived in the New World, the jury system was part of the English culture they brought to America. In October of 1765, representatives of nine colonies gathered in New York and published the Declaration of Rights, which was based on the common-law rights of Englishmen. One of the rights the colonists claimed in this Declaration was the right to trial by jury.

Thus began the jury system in the United States. As each colony was admitted as a state, each state made up a constitution and guaranteed the right to trial by jury – except Louisiana, which was governed by France before it was acquired by the United States. In conclusion, the jury system in the United States is the direct and comparable extension of the English jury.

The next question that came to my mind was, what is good about the system and what is bad. According to trial attorney Morris J. Bloomstein, there are many claims in which the use of a jury in all cases is wasteful of time and money. The most important claim against the jury system is that the quality of justice may be improved if trials were decided by a judge rather than by jurors. In my opinion, the whole question of the jury system can be reduced to the following question: Can twelve jurors bring better judgment than one judge or not?

In most cases, a mass of people shows a lower judgment than each person would show individually. For example, history tells us that in wartime many soldiers in many countries have killed innocent people, including babies and the old. Many people become violent when they are formed in groups, such as in student or racial riots. Individual people have conscience but a mass of people can be irrational. If this is the case, a group of jurors may decrease the quality of judgment. And, since jurors are no more intelligent than normal citizens, how can we expect the sum of these normal people's judgment to be better than that of a highly trained specialist of the law?

In my opinion, in the case of a small group of people such as a jury, individual judgment adds up to produce better and more balanced judgment than that of one person, even a highly educated judge. On this, Morris Bloomstein says in his book, *Verdict: The Jury System*, (Dodd, Mead, & Co., 1972), "With regard to the memories and intelligence of jurors, most trial attorneys find that jurors do not forget facts and legal instruction quite so easily. If one forgets, another remembers. It is the collective recollection and intelligence of the 12 panelists that counts, not that of any one juror."

Finally, the jury system is a democratic application of law practice. It is faith in ourselves instead of government and it is an expression of justice, which is something everyone has. This is a great system; we should keep it and develop it. Bloomstein writes, "Sir Patrick Devlin has called the jury 'the Lamp of Freedom'. May that lamp never be extinguished, for if darkness prevailed, further rights would surely be lost . . . As in the days of America's founding fathers, of Thomas Jefferson, of Patrick Henry, the jury remains the central pillar of the 'Temple of Justice', a pillar that must remain firm so that liberty may flourish."

The following incident shows the justice of the Englishmen who created the present jury system, again from Bloomstein's *Verdict*. As long as this spirit of justice exists, there is freedom of humanity.

> What is amazing, however, is that attaint was still applicable to juries up to 1670. At that time, two men who were being persecuted for their religious beliefs were brought to trial for unlawfully congregating with their co-religionists. Under the English statutes then prevailing, there was not a doubt that they were guilty, but with a sense of rebellion against the harshness of the law, the jury found the men not guilty. The entire jury was immediately held by the trial judge to be guilty of attaint. Riots erupted throughout England. Finally, on appeal, the entire concept of attaint was struck down. One of the two defendants was William Penn, founder of Pennsylvania.

In this sickness-ridden, economically unstable, war-feared, and crime-infested world, a group of people (in *The Verdict*) stood for justice. This movie shows hope for humanity, for as long as this justice exists in us, humanity will not die out. As Ohsawa said, the seventh condition of health is justice. As long as we have justice, we are healthy.

The Value of Salt

The macrobiotic diet never uses refined table salt but rather natural salt, as table salt is lacking many important minerals, especially trace minerals which are difficult to obtain from other foods. These trace minerals help enzymatic action for digestion and metabolism. Without these trace minerals, salt is a stimulant and can be dangerous for heart problems. Rather than using any table salt at all, we should use salt only in cooking or condiment form, combined with oil or other organic matter, so that our intestines can absorb it through the villi.

Using salt in cooking or grinding it with sesame seeds (to make *gomashio*, or sesame salt, for a table condiment) is the way to change salt to an organic form. This form of salt does not stimulate the nervous system as much as table salt does when salt passes through the blood vessels. It also does not stimulate the kidneys much, so it can penetrate inside the body to the intercellular and intracellular fluids. Then the organic matter separates from salt and the salt will be ionized and keep the inter- and intracellular fluids alkaline and yang. This means our nervous system, especially the interbrain, can maintain a steady state of its function. In other words, when those body fluids are yang and alkaline, our nervous and hormone systems maintain a balanced condition, even when we encounter bacteria or emotional difficulties.

In macrobiotic cooking, we recommend at least twenty minutes cooking after adding salt. This ensures that the salt will be combined with some organic matter such as oil, fat, or protein and in turn will also prevent a salty taste in the meals.

The common idea that salt causes water retention is misleading. Water retention is caused by osmosis existing between two liquids separated by a membrane. If the concentration of salt is higher in the blood plasma than the intercellular fluid, then water moves from intercellular fluid to blood plasma and to urine. In this case, we lose water. If the concentration of salt is lower in the plasma than the intercellular fluid, then water moves toward the intercellular fluids. In this case, we retain or gain water.

What causes the high concentration of salt in the intercellular and intracellular fluids is salt which came from the past diet. Such salt increases when we eat a lot of animal foods but not when eating grains or vegetables.

Therefore, if one has eaten cheese, meat, chicken, and so on for a long time, he or she retains water as well as fat. (This can result in obesity.) In other words, one who retains old salt cannot take much new salt. As a result he retains water, causing high blood pressure. He should eliminate old salt first. If one eliminates old salt and old fat, one will rejuvenate and increase health immediately. Without eliminating old salt, even the macrobiotic diet gives little benefit.

How can we eliminate old salt? Sweating helps, because along with sweat comes water with salt from tissue and muscles. This sweating brings another benefit: it also eliminates old fat, and one can reduce overweight by this method. How to sweat? Work hard physically. Laziness leads to fat and sickness. One who works hard maintains health and strength because he can consume the proper amount of salt. He can do this because he doesn't retain old salt. It is eliminated through sweating.

Now, in this civilized society, we sweat less and less. We cannot eliminate old salt and take new salt in. The old salt makes our tissues hard (yang) and our organs rigid, and the body ages quickly. Even ten minutes of sweating every day will rejuvenate a person ten years. Jogging, exercise, and saunas will bring sweat; however, the best way to sweat is through gardening, which will improve health and at the same time produce good foods.

Salt is the strongest alkaline-forming mineral. Therefore, vegetables cooked or aged by salt become strong alkaline-forming foods. Since many sicknesses are from an acidic condition, the proper use of salt will be a very good remedy for many sicknesses. In my opinion, cancer will not be controlled without the proper use of salt.

Salt gives strong energy and resistance against infections and bacterial diseases. One who likes salty food seems to me to have a strong immune system. When one stops eating animal foods, he must consume some salt. Otherwise he may end up with infectious diseases such as parasites, worms, or herpes, or he will be too introverted, docile, or alienated from society.

A macrobiotic student left my house to live by himself after having lived with us for about six months. When he visited a few months later he said our food had been too salty and too yang for him and that this had caused him to go out and eat ice cream often. Many Americans are like him, especially those who have eaten much animal food before starting the macrobiotic diet. They cannot eat salty foods or yang vegetables, even though these foods may not taste overly salty to other people, because they are retaining old salt.

There are three reasons, in my opinion, why some people cannot eat salty foods or why foods may be too salty for one person and not another. The first reason is that some people have this high salt content in their body cells and fluids due to a previous large consumption of animal foods. Because of this, the recent Japanese macrobiotic recommendation has been to take *shiitake* mushrooms (black Japanese mushrooms) or *konnyaku* (a gelatin-like cake made from yams) cooked with a little salt or no salt. We should have given our friend *shiitake* or *konnyaku* without soy sauce when he was staying in our home. However, he didn't tell us about this craving for ice cream until after he left.

A second reason may be weak kidneys. The kidney controls the amount of minerals in the body, especially sodium. If the kidneys are weak, excess sodium circulates in the blood and will cause much stimulation to the parasympathetic nerves; this causes thirst, and inhibition of the heart, kidney, liver, spleen, and pancreas functions which in turn can result in depression and dragging behavior.

The third reason one cannot take salty foods, or may think foods are salty even though they are not too salty for others, is a psychological one – that of judgment. When depression, hang-ups, cravings, dragginess, or other physical symptoms appear, a macrobiotic student usually thinks he is eating too yang or too salty. However, many times this is not true. Rather, he is too yin. In most cases the kidneys may be too weak to discharge the toxins and/or excess sodium. While the kidneys are failing to discharge the toxins and salts, these remain in the blood-stream, body fluids, and cells and cause physical reactions or psychological effects. Then a person thinks he is eating too salty or yang and may crave some yin foods. He tends to blame the foods but not his condition. He may not be aware of the need to repair his kidneys, and he may stop the symptoms of the kidney disease by taking yin food or drink. Therefore, the kidney condition does not improve but stays the same even if he has been on the diet for many years. The solution for such a case is very difficult. The person may blame and resent the diet or may give up the diet, thinking it is not right for him.

In order to avoid such trouble and prevent such unhappiness

from happening, we should teach the macrobiotic diet carefully. One solution for this would be not to give any quantities of ingredients in cookbooks so that everyone cooks by his or her own taste or need. Then when mistakes are made, we will have no one to blame but ourselves. This way of education is *dō*. It is one of the quickest ways to improve judgment. Since most Americans are not trained in this way, we give quantities for each ingredient mentioned in recipes. However, you should disregard the quantities after you have tried a recipe once or twice so that you will find the quantity best suited for you or your family.

Sodium and chlorides stay outside the cells and potassium and phosphates stay inside the cells, working together to maintain a balance which is essential to proper functioning of the cells and the organs they build. In the blood plasma, sodium helps maintain the proper acid-alkaline balance. Sodium also participates in conducting nerve impulses and thus affects muscle contractions.

Salt is highly important to the digestive process. In the gastric juices the chlorine of salt aids in the manufacture of hydrochloric acid, necessary for digestion in the stomach. Chlorine also becomes part of the extracellular tissue fluids in the body, as does sodium.

Salt also aids in the production of bile, which helps digestion in the intestines. Salt stimulates the peristaltic movement of the digestive tract and to a certain extent affects muscle strength.

Salt is a carrier for iodine. A small quantity of this element is needed to prevent goiter.

An important point in considering the poisonous potential of salt is the quantity of usage. Quantity changes quality. This simple law of nature, which has been taught by George Ohsawa, is so valid in all foods. Any food will be poisonous if we eat too much. Salt makes food delicious; without it foods are tasteless. Too much salt, however, can cause many poison-ous results, as Dr. Bieler (*Food Is Your Best Medicine*, Random House, 1973) has said. But if we say only that salt is poisonous, it is too hasty a conclusion. Arsenic is a good medicine for syphilis if used in the proper quantity. However, it also has been one of the strongest poisons in history.

Poisons and medicines are the front and back. Sickness and health, bad and good, ugliness and beauty are all front and back. They are the two sides of Oneness. There are no foods without these two characteristics. Therefore, all natural food is medicine and can be poison at the same time. However, unnat-ural chemical food products are always poisonous (one side only) because they lack the natural order. The French scientist Kervran formulated a hypothesis called 'biological atomic transmutation'. If we accept this concept, old sodium accumu-lated from animal foods over a long period of time can be changed to potassium by the following equation. The number shows the atomic weight of each element.

$$Na^{23} + O^{16} \rightarrow K^{39}$$

This transmutation, however, only occurs if one does hard exercise such as to induce heavy sweating. In such a case, sodium becomes extremely yang and fuses with yin oxygen so hard that it changes even the nucleus. Such transmutation does not occur in normal activities.

As I mentioned earlier, trace minerals are very important in the metabolism of salt. However, most salt sold at the market is lacking trace minerals. Therefore, it is not utilized in our body but passes through the alimentary canal serving as a stimulant. This kind of salt is overconsumed and may be hazardous to our health.

It seems to me that among most people suffering from hypertension who have reduced their blood pressure by taking less salt, most are heavy animal food eaters. Their arteries are clogged by cholesterol and they have too much old salt in their tissues, making their muscles and arteries stiff. Consequently less salt, no salt, or salt substitutes by potassium will bring comfort for their hypertension. However, sticking to a no-salt diet for a long time will create a sodium-deficient condition. I met several such persons recently. They are easily tired, their hands and legs are cold, and they often have leg cramps.

There are a few people in this country conscious enough to make good salt or to import natural sea salt from abroad. This salt is much more expensive, but healthwise it will save money in the long run. Such people are Naboru Muramoto and Jacques deLangre. I am not interested in recommending any particular product, but either of these would be a much better salt than the normal salt sold at the market.

The Second Time

Ms. C. cured her sickness following the macrobiotic diet faithfully about four years ago. She became very healthy. She enjoyed her diet, but it was too rigid. She started to binge. According to her letter, around March of 1982 she started to binge a little and then a lot. She would go out to lunch almost every day and have poached eggs on toast and two to three cups of coffee. Sometimes she had a turkey sandwich. She also had cheese and biscuits at night if she had a craving for cheese, although she normally didn't like dairy products.

In October she began to lose weight and developed a burning in the mouth and genitals. Then she stayed with the grain and vegetable diet again, strictly, but the situation didn't improve. She started worrying and wondering.

She wrote me a handwritten letter, but it was written so badly I couldn't read it. I kept the letter on my desk in the 'to be answered' file for two or three weeks. As she didn't get an answer from me she started asking several people. Each gave different answers or advice, so she was more confused.

At this stage, she wrote me another letter, typewritten. Then it was time for me to think. Why did she cure her sickness so easily the first time but not the second time? I have observed similar cases many times among my macrobiotic friends. Mr. O. cured cancer with macrobiotics, but he started to binge almost seven years after he started the diet. The cancer became active again. This time he couldn't cure it and he died. Mr. N. cured cancer by the diet almost twenty years ago; then he started eating very badly on occasion, the cancer returned, and he soon died.

While I was thinking about this, a letter came from Japan saying that an older macrobiotic leader had just died. He was almost eighty so he was old enough, but he could have lived longer. Reflecting on his death, I understood the so-called mystery of the macrobiotic diet.

People who cure their sickness by the diet often do not cure completely; some toxins or disturbed parts of organs remain. This sickness doesn't show or come out because good foods cover things up. However, as one starts eating badly the toxins are helped to be powerful agents once more, causing ill symptoms. The toxins are much worse and stronger than the first time because the illness has gone much deeper. Therefore, one who tries to cure a second time experiences more difficulties. At this time people start wondering and ask several opinions. Receiving different advice from different people, they are confused and will worry more. Sickness progresses.

The most important thing is to have faith in the diet. And from this faith must come a real understanding of macrobiotics.

Ms. C. cured her sickness four years ago but she never studied macrobiotic philosophy and principles. Therefore, she had difficulties when she was sick the second time. I am responsible for this. Instead of teaching her the principles so that she could cure sicknesses by herself, or at least not be upset and unable to handle them, I taught her only the diet.

Postscript: I received a letter from her friend saying that she is better now.

April 1983

Gandhi

You should see the movie called *Gandhi*. It will give you one of the biggest spiritual inspirations in your life, as well as deep doubt concerning human nature because even Gandhi's greatness couldn't cure the human sickness of violence. However, before seeing the movie, you must read Gandhi's autobiography. Here, for your reference, I write an introductory note on what I learned from French writer Romain Rolland's *Mahatma Gandhi* (Garland Publishing, 1973) and George Ohsawa's *Eternal Youth* (not available in English).

During his whole life Gandhi pursued the attainment of truth inside himself, and fought the injustice of the British government outside himself. His weapon was 'noncooperation and nonviolence'. Gandhi probably learned this from the 'civil disobedience' of Thoreau and Tolstoy. The tactics of noncooperation had been defined by Gandhi and the committee of noncooperation, including:

> Surrender of all the titles of honorary office.
> Boycott of English government schools.
> Nonparticipation in English government parties and
>   other official functions.
> Refusal to accept any civil or military posts. (Is this
>   the origin of conscientious objection?)
> Spreading the doctrine of Swadeshi. (Swadeshi:

Swa, self or oneself; Deshi, country. Hence, national
independence. The noncooperators usually interpreted
it in the narrower sense of economic independence.)
American industrial leaders in the 1980s are following
Gandhi by boycotting Japanese goods in order to sustain their industries.

Gandhi preached Swadeshi only in order to establish India's
economic independence. His first practice of Swadeshi was to
boycott European wine. He begged the liquor dealers to stop
selling alcohol. All India responded to Gandhi's appeal, but so
many crowds started destroying the wine shops and closing
them by force that Gandhi had to tell them, "You must not try
to compel another by physical force."

The next step of Gandhi's Swadeshi was giving up imported
cotton clothes; instead, he encouraged Indians to use their
leisure hours for spinning cloth. Romain Rolland explains,
"Eighty percent of the population of India is agricultural, and
is therefore without employment virtually four months of the
year. One-tenth of the population is normally exposed to
famine . . . . India, who grows all the cotton she requires, is
forced to export millions of bales to Japan and Lancashire,
whence it is returned to her in the form of manufactured calico,
which she must buy at exorbitant prices." Therefore, Gandhi's first plan was to organize workshops to create employment and feed her people. Such workshops urged people to
spin and weave at home. Gandhi said spinning was a duty for
all India. He wanted everyone, man and woman, to contribute
at least one hour a day to spinning. He even taught precise
techniques of spinning and weaving. Hindu and Moslem
women agreed to wear only domestically-made clothes, which
became the fashion.

However, Gandhi did go too far in ordering the burning of
all foreign goods in Bombay in August 1921. According to Rolland, Gandhi explained this action as follows: "The materials

were not burned as an expression of hatred for England, but as a sign of India's determination to break with the past. It was a necessary surgical operation." This action caused disputes among intellectuals who had been supporters of the noncooperation movement.

As Gandhi's main purpose was to unite India – that is to say, unite all religions, races, parties, and castes – he thought the teaching of unity was important, and he founded the school called Satyagrah Ashram (ashram means place of discipline). The character of this ashram was unique because it was concerned with the teachers more than the students. The teachers had to take the following vows:

The vow of truth: This is extremely similar to Ohsawa's seventh condition of health, which is honesty and justice. Ohsawa considered that being honest at all times is the most important sign of health, happiness, and greatness. Ohsawa most admired Gandhi because of his honesty.

The vow of Ahimsa (non-killing): Many vegetarians began their vegetarianism because of this; however, they do not realize that if they take antibiotic pills or chemotherapy drugs they are violating this vow.

The vow of celibacy: This is not a vow of the unmarried, but means if a man is married he will consider his wife a lifelong friend. Do not relate with the other sex only physically, without high spiritual ideals, respect, and commitment.

The control of the palate: Gandhi was a champion of the macrobiotic diet because he ate grains and vegetables, in small amounts, throughout his life. He vowed not to drink even cow's milk because it was against the vow of Ahimsa. He self-reflected deeply and confessed how he suffered when he ate meat.

The vow of non-stealing: Ohsawa used to say to us that it is stealing if we possess extra clothes, houses, or even foods more than we need; we stole them even if we think we paid their cost. For example, if we eat an apple every day we are stealing another's apple because apples are not produced enough to supply the earth's whole population. The same is true for animal foods. The rich pay a high price for meats and the poor can't buy them. We do not consider this stealing, but in Gandhi's sense this is so.

The vow of nonpossession: One of the macrobiotic principles Ohsawa taught was to live with only absolutely necessary things. So around the beginning of the 1970s many hippies left home and tried to live without possessions. Now, many young Americans join such things as Rev. Moon's church, throwing out their possessions. American parents as well as Eastern gurus don't understand that nonpossession is a virtue in the East but a crazy thing in the West.

Many idealists tried in vain to establish communities with this principle. There is one community in Japan which has been successfully following this principle for over eighty years called Itto-En, founded by Tenko Nishida. One who lives in this community does not possess anything. Everything is owned by the community.

The vow of Swadeshi: Gandhi taught not to use manufactured articles or foreign goods. Macrobiotic principles teach the eating of locally-grown and seasonal foods. Ohsawa's last macrobiotic advice was to establish a macrobiotic foods manufacturer within every 250-mile radius. In other words, we should observe Swadeshi in eating.

The vow of fearlessness: According to Ohsawa, one who has absolute faith in God (the order of the universe) has no fear. Therefore he is honest. Thus, fearlessness is in the character of one who attains supreme judgment.

The Satyagrah Ashram's uniqueness was not only in the teachers' vows but also the student regulations:

> Students were admitted at any age; however, they had
> to remain in the ashram for the whole course of studies,
> which lasted about ten years.

The students were separated from and did not visit their
parents.

The students wore simple clothes and ate simple,
strictly vegetarian meals.

No holidays, although once a week they had a day and a
half for individual creative work.

Students travelled on foot through India three months
of the year.

All students studied the Hindu and Dravidian dialects
as well as the five written Indian languages, with English as a second language.

They learned agriculture, spinning, and weaving as well
as history, geography, mathematics, economics, and
Sanskrit.

The tuition was free.

Gandhi considered this system the mainspring of the whole
movement. Gandhi was a powerful man as a political and
spiritual leader in 1921. People looked up to him as a saint. He
was the greatest leader India ever had in her history.

The bigger the front, the bigger the back is the order of the
universe. Gandhi's front was his great success as a leader. His
back was the theoretical opposition made by Rabindranath
Tagore. Tagore was not only a poet but he considered himself
Asia's spiritual ambassador to Europe. He had just returned
from Europe where he had asked people to cooperate in creating a world university at Santiniketan. The noncooperation of
Gandhi clashed with his way of thinking, his mentality, and his
intelligence which had been nourished by all cultures of the
world.

Gandhi tried to unite India through the negation of England. To Tagore this was contradictory. For him, unity is that
which embraces and understands everything; consequently it
cannot be attained through negation. Tagore thought the present age has been dominated by the Occident because the

Occident had a mission to fulfill. We of the Orient should learn from the Occident. Lacking this thinking, Japan started World War II and was defeated. After being defeated, Japan tried to learn from the West by all means. Japan mastered Western technology better than the West and made the greatest economic comeback of the world.

If we want to count any shortcoming of the great Gandhi, it would be his excluding Western civilization – while Tagore refused to negate Western civilization. Tagore feared the development of the spirit of exclusion. Tagore did not fear Gandhi but he feared the Gandhists who blindly followed Gandhi's nonviolent anti-English movement. In fact, such exclusive mentality eventually created the anti-Moslem or anti-Hindu mentality among Indians. This was Gandhi's biggest disillusionment and led finally to his death.

Gandhi himself had no exclusivity at all, and used it only as a tactic for the recovery of India. But this tactic destroyed both India and Gandhi. Ohsawa, therefore, taught us to never be exclusive.

According to Ohsawa, the most important lesson and the greatest virtue of Gandhi was his self-reflection. Gandhi probably accomplished a greater job than Buddha or Christ. However, his greatness was neither his political accomplishments nor his saintliness, but his self-reflection and honesty. Gandhi always considered himself a liar, a vow-breaker, and a non-virtuous man. Ironically, one who thinks himself ignorant or a great sinner is often the greatest man. Gandhi was such a great man. He always considered that it was his fault whenever Indians committed any violent acts, and he would start to purify his spirit by fasting. He fasted because he thought his spirit dirty and ugly. Such self-reflection moved 300 million Indians without the use of power or money.

Gandhi said, "Without self-reflection and self-cleansing, it is impossible to realize a man of universal being."

The Art of Binging

In macrobiotics, even binging must bring happiness. In order for this to happen, we have to learn the art of binging. What is the art of binging? First of all, we must not feel guilty when we do binge, because guilt feelings bring more damage to our lives than the binge itself does.

At the beginning of macrobiotic teaching in this country, people secretly went to restaurants so that other macrobiotic followers would not see them eating 'outside' foods. If they found other ones there, they were ashamed. Being ashamed is all right; however, people often feel guilty. This is not good because feelings of guilt make us miserable.

Gandhi ate meat against his vow. He felt guilty about this for a long time, because he broke his commitment made to God that he would not eat meat. Instead of feeling guilty, he could have just felt ashamed of being weak in not keeping his promise. In my opinion he shouldn't have felt guilty, because guilt is dualism. One who lives with God or the order of the universe has no guilt feelings. Guilt feelings come when we separate ourselves from oneness, God, or the order of the universe. (However, it is difficult to reach this mentality, so don't feel guilty if you have guilt feelings.)

Another reason to have feelings of guilt is eating too-yin foods. Eat fewer yin foods such as sugary foods, cakes, refreshing drinks, coffee, vinegar, alcohol, fruits, etc. In the art of binging, this comes first.

The next technique is that we should not binge alone, but with friends. By doing this, we can control the amount. If we binge by ourselves, we do so in greater quantities, but if we binge with others, we will not go to such an extreme because we are more conscious than when alone.

Third, we shouldn't eat any three extremes – either yin or yang – consecutively. In other words, we can eat ice cream and coffee, but not ice cream and coffee and fruits (as an example). We can eat fish and miso soup, but not fish, miso soup, and cheese.

Fourth, don't eat extreme yin or oily foods three days consecutively. This winter I went to Los Angeles on a lecture trip. After two days lecturing, I visited a health food convention where I ate at a restaurant three nights consecutively, with cheesecake for dessert. When I was lecturing at San Diego, I was losing my voice from too much cheesecake. It took almost one week for me to become normal after eating cheesecake three times. If I had eaten it only two nights in a row, I would not have been sick. I will not eat cheesecake for three nights consecutively again.

If you have to eat at a party or meeting, don't be afraid to binge. One meal will not kill you. You would do better to keep a friend than keep a diet. The diet is important, but a too-rigid mentality in trying to stay on the diet is not advisable. Even though we are observing a diet, we should maintain flexibility.

If you follow the art of binging, you will suffer less.

From Thinking
To Judgment

The macrobiotics which you are studying or are going to study includes an old way of eating. However, it was forgotten in the history of mankind; therefore, it is new to most people, in the East as well as the West. There is another aspect to macrobiotics, which is a way of thinking. The way of thinking practiced in macrobiotics is old. Like the macrobiotic diet, macrobiotic thinking is also lost; this is partly the result of so-called school education, because conventional school education is destructive to man's intuition or natural thinking.

What is unconventional thinking? The following story will illustrate:

Some time ago, an American shoe company sent two salesmen to Africa to investigate the possibility of shoe sales in Africa. One salesman reported to the company, "There is no possibility of sales because nobody in black Africa is wearing shoes." The other salesman said, "There is tremendous sales potential because nobody is wearing shoes yet." The first salesman's opinion is conventional thinking and the latter is unconventional thinking.

There is always conventional thinking and unconventional thinking. In most cases, conventional thinking was once unconventional.

When Nicholas Copernicus wrote *Concerning the Revolution of the Heavenly Bodies,* conventional thinking was that the earth is at rest in the center of the universe. But he suggested the possibility of the earth's turning around the sun. This was completely unconventional thinking. Observing the motion of the planets by a telescope, Galileo Galilei proved that the earth turns around the sun. Now, it is conventional thought that the earth rotates around the sun. Among these two revolutionary thinkers, Copernicus was a more unconventional and creative thinker while Galileo was a conventional and logical thinker.

When conventional thinking finds it impossible to solve problems, unconventional thinking may be the only answer. Most scientific theories are formed by unconventional thinking; many scientists have solved problems this way when they could not solve the problems by the conventional ways of thinking.

When Einstein made his famous Theory of Relativity, he did no experiments. What Einstein did was to check all information concerning Newtonian structure which was conventionally considered perfect and put the concept of relativity into it. This was unconventional thinking.

There is a very good book called *New Think* written by Edward de Bono (Basic Books, Inc., 1968) in which two types of thinking are discussed. One is called 'vertical thinking' and the other is 'lateral thinking'. According to de Bono:

> Vertical thinking has always been the only respectable type of thinking. Computers are perhaps the best example. The problem is defined by the programmer, who also indicates the path along which the problem is to be explored. The computer then proceeds with its incomparable logic and efficiency to work out the problem.
>
> Just as water flows down slopes, settles in hollows and is confined to riverbeds, so vertical thinking flows along the most probable paths and by its very flow increases the probability of those paths for the future.

Lateral thinking is easiest to appreciate when it is seen in action. Everyone has come across the sort of problem which seems impossible to solve until suddenly a surprisingly simple solution is revealed. Once it has been thought of, the solution is so obvious that one cannot understand why it was ever so difficult to find.

If vertical thinking is high-probability thinking, then lateral thinking is low-probability thinking. New channels are deliberately cut to alter the flow of the water. The old channels are dammed up in the hope that the water will seek out and take to new and better patterns of flow. When the low-probability line of thought leads to an effective new idea there's a 'eureka moment', and at once the low-probability approach acquires the highest probability. It is the moment when the water sucked upward with difficulty forms a siphon and at once flows freely. This moment is always the aim of lateral thinking.

In short, vertical thinking is putting up the toy blocks one by one. One must carefully put one block on top of another. However, in the case of lateral thinking, the blocks are placed without order or pattern.

The important message we get from *New Think* is that one must think from both sides if he wants to be creative and free and overcome difficulties. Dr. de Bono teaches how to think laterally. It requires discipline and exercise.

In the Orient, techniques for thinking have been developed. That is yin and yang thinking. We can develop unconventional (lateral) thinking by learning yin and yang thinking. Columbus sailed west and found the West Indies. If he had sailed east he may have found India as he planned at first. Thus one can always find two ways in thinking and action.

After hundreds of experiments, scientists have found that the two halves of our brain work in distinctly different ways. The left brain thinks logically, while the right brain is good for shapes and images. Watching TV may strengthen the right brain but maybe not the left brain. Therefore, the new generation will be good at video games but may not be good at philosophy.

With yin and yang thinking, such a distinction is apparent because the left side is yin and the right side is yang. Without knowing modern science, we can imagine the difference between the left and right brain if we know the qualities of yin and yang.

Yin and yang thinking advises us that we must think always one way and then its opposite; then our thinking becomes more complete or full. Our thinking tends to be one-sided because we use one side of the brain more than the other. In a sense, the yin and yang concept gives us tremendous freedom of thinking if we learn this properly.

An important characteristic of macrobiotic thinking is its paradoxical thinking. Paradoxical thinking is Oriental thinking and it was named so by the famous psychologist, Erich Fromm. According to Fromm, there are two kinds of logic which make two kinds of thinking. One is Aristotelian thinking and logic and the other is paradoxical thinking which is based on paradoxical logic.

Aristotelian logic is based on the law of identity (A is A), the law of contradiction (A is not non-A), and the law of the excluded middle (X cannot be A and non-A at the same time).

This logic is the foundation of Western scientific thinking. However, in *The Art of Loving* (Harper & Row, 1974), Fromm says: "This axiom of Aristotelian logic has so deeply imbued our habits of thought that it is felt to be natural and self-evident, while on the other hand the statement that X is A and not A at the same time seems to be nonsensical."

For simple-minded persons, without deep thinking, the statement "A is A" is valid. But from the careful observation of the world and our experiences, it is obvious that there is no A in existence which is identical to another A. In other words, "A is A" is imaginary thinking, not realistic, because A is always changing. A is no more A at the next second. Such thinking is paradoxical thinking which is well expressed by the teaching of Lao Tsu, Buddha, and other Oriental wise men.

George Ohsawa called this paradoxical thinking 'supreme judgment'. In his seven stages of judgment, it can be seen as the last, or the first.

Seventh stage judgment: Supreme judgment can be described as follows:

1. There is nothing identical. This is the negation of the law of identity and is valid always and anywhere. So this is truth, and the supreme judgment.

2. That which has a beginning has an end. (A → non-A). This is the negation of the law of contradiction. It also can be said that everything changes. 'Everything changes' has been a basic concept in India, China, and Japan. One of the greatest poets of China, Ri Tei Pei, wrote: "The whole universe is a hotel in which all matter stops over; / Time is a passenger which passes by through the dream of life."

A famous Japanese poet, Basho, begins his Haiku book *Okuno Hosomichi* by saying that ". . . our life is nothing but a journey. Some will travel by horse, some by boat and some on foot. In any event, everything is a journey. In old age, the journey itself becomes the resting place." In other words, 'everything changes' does not change. Therefore, this is truth – the supreme judgment.

3. That which has a front has a back. This is the negation of the law of the excluded middle. In figure 1, A is the front of the coin X, and non-A is the back of the coin X. Therefore, A and non-A are nothing but the manifestation of the same X. Therefore, X does not exclude A and non-A.

Another example of an explanation of the negation of the law

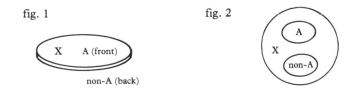

fig. 1

X   A (front)

non-A (back)

fig. 2

A

X

non-A

of the excluded middle is figure 2 in which X can be A and non-A at the same time. A and non-A represent all matter and phenomena, and X is totality, infinity, or the origin of all matter and phenomena (or oneness, the 'tao' of Lao Tsu). In other words, infinity or oneness does not exclude the middle. This is also the supreme judgment.

From the viewpoint of macrobiotics, Aristotelian thinking (law of identity, law of contradiction, and law of excluded middle) is static and therefore valid only when it is applied in a limited and partial way. In other words, Aristotelian thinking does not lead us to eternal truth. Therefore, judgment based on this logic leads us to antagonism and war. On the contrary, paradoxical thinking (such as that of Erich Fromm) leads us to truth. This is thinking by the supreme judgment.

Aristotelian thinking or judgment will not embrace A with non-A, yin with yang, right with wrong, rich with poor, black with white, and vice versa; rather, these will antagonize each other. Therefore, Aristotelian thinking is the thinking of antagonism, separation, and alienation. No wonder that Western mentality, superstitiously believing in the Aristotelian form of logic, has led the world to antagonism, hatred, war, violence, and crime. Contrary to Aristotelian thinking, supreme judgment is the thinking of truth and is all-embracing. Therefore, it can explain and understand totality. It can be applied from the changing world to eternity or infinity.

Ohsawa called A and non-A yin and yang. Here, yin is not

absolutely yin but a yin and yang accumulation with yin dominating. In the same way, yang is not absolutely yang but it is an accumulation of yin and yang where yang dominates.

Like front and back, yin and yang are two sides of X (infinity or oneness). Simply, we can say that yin and yang are the two sides of infinity.

The above can be stated as follows: infinity polarizes itself into yin and yang. This is the emergence of yin and yang. From this yin and yang all things and phenomena are created. Ohsawa called supreme judgment 'the order of the universe'. The relationship between supreme judgment and the order of the universe can be explained as follows: supreme judgment is consciousness of infinity, while the order of the universe is the constitution of infinity.

Since supreme judgment is the consciousness of infinity, or infinity itself, it is perfect, true, and all-embracing love. It exists anywhere and anytime. It is like a radio wave or TV wave. It exists in the air but we don't know if we don't tune it in. Other lower judgments are also like radio waves, not only supreme judgment.

As infinity descends to the levels of yin and yang, energy, pre-atoms, elements, and plants and animals, supreme or seventh stage judgment also descends. It manifests lower judgments because lower judgment is a part of high judgment.

Sixth stage judgment: The judgment of ideologies is next to supreme judgment. Human nature is good or bad; man is sinful or not; this world is wonderful, beautiful or this world is suffering; materialism and spiritualism – all belong to this stage of judgment.

Fifth stage judgment: From ideological judgment, the social, religious, and economical judgments appear because ideological judgment includes social judgment. For example, the judgment which thinks "man's nature is good" produces religions such as Shinto and the Nichiren sect; the judgment which thinks "man is sinful" creates religions such as Christianity and the Shin sect of Buddhism, etc.

Economic judgment creates systems of economy such as communism and capitalism. This is another part of the fifth judgment.

Fourth stage judgment: From social and religious judgment comes intellectual judgment (rational and artistic). It forms various scientific concepts, ideas, and theories. Also, social and religious concepts influence art, music, and literature, which are the artistic expression of intellectual judgment.

Third stage judgment: From intellectual, rational, and artistic judgment emotional judgment appears, such as like and dislike, joy or sadness, satisfaction or complaint.

Second stage judgment: Sensorial judgment includes sense perceptions such as color, sound, temperature, shape, touch, etc.

First stage judgment: Finally, autonomic nervous action; the mechanical or intuitive function of consciousness manifests.

Judgment thus encompasses from oneness to intuition. However, its realization requires the individual body. In other words, certain conditions are necessary for the human body or animals to manifest either intuitive autonomic mechanical judgment as seen in unicellular organisms or the sensorial judgment seen in fishes and all animals.

A highly developed person can manifest his or her judgment at will such as intellectual, social, religious, and ideological.

The freest and happiest person is one who can manifest supreme judgment – all-embracing love and absolute justice.

Everyone is receiving such judgment. However, the level of judgment that will be tuned in and appear on our screen of life depends on our constitution and physical condition. In order to perceive higher stages of judgment, we need to always improve our physical and spiritual condition. Right diet, meditation, proper exercises, chanting, etc., are disciplines by which we can improve our perceptions.

Prayer is nothing but calling for the spiritual vibration to come to us so that we are able to perceive clearly.

Judgment of infinity thus contains seven stages of judgment from mechanical, intuitive judgment to supreme judgment. At the time of birth, we have mechanical and intuitive judgment. After some days, we have sensorial judgments which perceive temperatures, color, shapes, etc.

After some months, we have like and dislike – sentimental judgment. In the fourth stage, we can explain things logically and distinguish phenomena. As we further develop to the fifth stage, we create religions such as Buddhism and Christianity, and economic systems such as capitalism and communism.

In the sixth stage, ideology develops (dualism, materialism, spiritualism, life's affirmation or negation, etc.).

In the seventh stage, our judgment is supreme, our consciousness is infinite. It is all-embracing love and judgment, with no antagonism. Supreme judgment exists here and now all the time. However, whether we are able to manifest the judgment of truth, love, and happiness depends on our condition and constitution.

"In any case, we cannot possess supreme judgment from the very beginning," wrote Ohsawa in *The Book of Judgment*. "We must first develop the lower judgment. Therefore, we must endure heat, cold, hunger and the greatest difficulties not only in childhood, but during one's entire life. And as one grows older, life seems more full of difficulties and sadness. We love and are betrayed. We are often desperate. Without having lived such a life, we cannot develop our judgment." After passing difficulties, sadness, joy, and argumentations, we reach sixth and finally seventh judgment.

The first to sixth judgments are the roots of seventh

judgment. We should not eliminate lower judgments because without them there is no supreme judgment. However, we will not be able to be happy without reaching the seventh, supreme judgment. For this we must observe right diet, meditation, chanting, and proper exercises. The most important thing is that we must make a commitment to ourselves:

> We will not exclude anyone or anything, even cancer, from our list of friends.
> We will accept all difficulties with greatest pleasure, even one who hates us.
> We will not complain whenever we receive misfortune or unfair treatment.
> We will keep our promises by all means.
> We will not lie.
> We will say thank you even for betrayals, disloyalties, and hatred.
> We will consider that all things and people are one.

When we are able to realize even one of these commitments, we have reached supreme judgment.

How To Overcome Fear
From a lecture at Vega

Fear is an issue in almost everyone's life today and there are some basic tools we can use to help overcome it.

The first ones deal with the physiological aspect of oneself, the body, and have to do with what one consumes. To overcome fear, one should eat no sugar; sugar encourages fear. If you don't eat any sugar, you have taken the first big step towards being free from fear. The next is to drink less. Fear is related to poorly functioning kidneys, and restricting liquids eases the burden on them. If you drink more you will fear more, worry more. When you consume less liquid the kidneys function more efficiently and you have less fear, less worry. Interestingly, you can effect this change immediately. If you don't drink much for one day your fear will diminish. Very, very simple.

The next tool is psychological and addresses the more spiritual aspects of oneself. This is more difficult, needing more understanding. You need the understanding of universal law, of macrobiotics. First of all you have to use your will to make a commitment: "I am going to cure my disease." You must make this commitment yourself. This step helps overcome fear because as soon as you make a commitment you become a different person. The commitment you make doesn't come from yourself, it comes from outside yourself, from the 'big Self' or universal Self. There is no fear involved, only a calm, clear understanding. Commitment then is made by the big Self, and the small self (what you normally identify with, the ego or conscious mind) is only a receiver. How clear you are in your understanding of the fact that you are but a part of the larger Self is the measure of your success or defeat. If your understanding is very clear you can overcome any difficulty. All difficulties, whether cancer or just an uncontrollable urge to eat ice cream, are rooted in one's identifying with the small self and not the Self.

Each morning at our Vega study house we do some chanting – the *Hannya Shin Gyo*; we are talking about this Self. In the field of psychology they work with the small self and try to help one overcome it, but they don't give you the information to put you in touch with the Self. You have to overcome the small self to reach the true Self. What brings the big Self and the small self together is called *hannya* in Chinese or Sanskrit. What does *hannya* mean? The small self reaching the big Self or oneness. When we finally reach it and merge with it, we have no more fear or worry. Trying to reach the higher Self is the goal of Eastern training, Eastern discipline. Japanese samurai must go through rigorous training, and the most important aspect is reaching the Self. When they reach oneness, they are no longer afraid of fighting. When we identify with the small self we are afraid, "Oh, he is going to kill me." We are always afraid someday someone stronger will attack us. As long as we identify with our small self, fear and worry are unavoidable.

It's the same thing, whether you have good health or a million dollars, you worry that somehow it will be taken away. If you identify with the small self, even if you are very, very healthy, you will always worry that someday you will somehow lose that health. And if you are very sick and you identify with this self, you will also always worry – "I am going to die soon, I'll never be cured." But if you know the Self, then there is no worry. Why? Because the Self is eternal. The self is temporal, short-lived – usually eighty years at the most, maybe only fifty years. That is what we are clinging to. We are seeing only it, feeling only it. We are clinging, attached. We think we are the self, we have been told we are. That's the mistake of our current educational system.

I was born in southern Japan and when I was nine years old I was sent to Tokyo to be adopted by my uncle and his wife. They had no children, so they took me in as their son. My parents had ten children which was too many to support; they were poor. The countryside where I was born was very quiet – so yin. I grew up very yin. Then I went to Tokyo, which was the center of industry. Next to my house was a factory – ga-tang, ga-tang, ga-tang. There was so much yang movement and noise, and my adopted mother gave me fish two times a day, fish at every meal. I became more and more yang. So I inherited a yin constitution and acquired a yang condition. Two extremes, fighting each other within me. I could not decide on a course of action. One day I would want to do something one way and the next morning I would want to do it a different way – very schizophrenic. For a long time I suffered with this schizophrenic mentality because of those radical changes in my diet and environment. Very, very sad.

When I was finished with school I began chasing girls – dance floor girls or prostitutes. When the American forces first came to Japan, the first thing they did was to build dance halls as entertainment for the soldiers. I used to go to them to chase girls. That was the result of the change in my condition, though I didn't know it. Deep inside I was more spiritual but outside I just wanted to chase girls, so my uncle worried very much. He thought I should get married, so he selected a girl and I said okay. This caused big problems because we moved in with my adoptive parents, and my adopted mother and my new wife couldn't get along living together. My wife wasn't happy. I didn't know it but she wasn't happy at all; she didn't say anything to me. One day she just left home and took an overdose of sleeping pills to commit suicide. She was found dead a few months later. I was so disturbed I lost my mind. The only thing I could think of to do was go to Ohsawa's school. Somehow I had to find out how to live, so I went.

There were about twenty to thirty students at that time, and the students were expected to help out doing the jobs that needed to be done, such as publishing a magazine and selling it on the streets, cleaning the house, etc. I couldn't do anything. I had lost my mind. All I did was eat, sleep, and attend Ohsawa's lectures. That was all I could do, nothing else. But those lectures meant life and death to me. I had to understand so I could live again. So I listened carefully and Ohsawa said many things. I didn't move any tables or bring any food; I didn't do anything but listen to his lectures. For one month I listened very, very attentively – one month.

At the end of the month I understood. I understood that I am not the small self but a part of the larger Self. Individual cells make up the whole body but each individual cell is unique, separated by a membrane from each other and making up the community of our body. Our bodies are also separated by a membrane called skin and we live in communities that make up humanity on Earth. And maybe our planet, separated by its atmospheric skin, combines with others forming communities which then make up the whole universe. Individuals, whether cells or people, are separated by a membrane, but in reality we are all one.

In the process of thinking you are identifying with your small self, but actually the universal Self is thinking and the small self or brain is receiving, like a TV set. The signals in vibrational form come in from infinity from all directions, and your brain receives these signals. So worry comes in from the outside, fear and joy too. But what kind of signal do you receive? The kind of signal you choose depends on the condition of your receiver. All the signals are surrounding you – joy surrounds you, happiness surrounds you, worry surrounds you; all the possibilities are there. The signals are everywhere all the time. However, even though you have a TV set, until you switch it on you aren't aware of which channel it is set on. But as soon as you turn it on you can tune the channel to the station you want. Some show a happy story, some show a very sad story. It's up to you what you pull in, what you select. It's all up to you. You are entitled to choose any channel, that is your free will. If you want to live a sad story you can choose so, but if you want a happy life, that is there too. All the signals surround us and the small self chooses.

If you eat more grain and vegetables, drink less, and do not eat sugar, you will attract less fear. That is what I learned when I was in Ohsawa's school. He didn't teach how to make an albi plaster or how to make a ginger compress. He didn't teach how to eat or how to choose food. He didn't teach what food is yin and what food is yang. He never even taught how to cook; sometimes the food there was lousy. I didn't like it very much. In Japan we never learned about yin and yang. After I came to America I learned these other things – Michio too. After we came here we taught ourselves. But I learned one thing from Ohsawa, that the Self is the real me. It is the real you. Individuals are separate, they look different, right? But the source of all individuality is one – the big Self. To me this was the biggest finding, the most joyful thing I had ever known. I found that all people are the same, that all are my brothers and sisters. I found my neighbors the same as me. Americans looked different when I came here but I found them the same as me too, some more yin and some more yang, but still of the same oneness.

As you begin to understand this, fear gradually goes away; and when you clearly understand this, fear is gone. You have to understand this to really overcome fear. This is called reaching God. This is totality, consciousness – universal consciousness, or oneness. When you clearly understand what is your real Self and what is your temporal self, there is no fear.

Ohsawa's Most Important Concept

To most people, George Ohsawa is the founder of the macrobiotic diet, which is based on whole grains. Twenty years have passed since he first lectured on macrobiotics in this country. His diet has been condemned as the most dangerous diet, public enemy number one, by some medical doctors. Under such condemnation the macrobiotic diet has been supported all these years by many followers until, finally, scientific nutritional thinking has gradually changed. Recent trends in nutrition or diets for health (the U.S. Dietary Goals, the Pritikin Diet) are now very similar to the macrobiotic approach. In my opinion, as science develops, the macrobiotic diet will prove its superiority as a human health diet.

This is one of Ohsawa's great contributions to the world. However, he made many more important contributions. That is to say, his explanation of the mind – memory, thinking, and the mechanism of thinking – is far more important than the diet. In my opinion, his concept of these is much clearer than that of Buddha, Christ, Confucius, and even Lao Tsu.

However, I couldn't find his writings on this concept except in Japanese. I checked *Zen Macrobiotics* (Ohsawa Foundation, 1965), *The Unique Principle* (G.O.M.F., 1976), and *The Atomic Age* (G.O.M.F., 1977) in vain to find at least partial explanations. Yet, he discussed and explained these things in his lectures all the time. In fact, he rarely spoke of diet. One of my friends, an American lawyer, said one day after attending several of his lectures, "This (concept) is extraordinary."

Therefore, those who did not attend his lectures will have missed one of the most important concepts they could have. I feel it is my duty to make this information available to Americans and others who did not attend his lectures.

What is the most important concept George Ohsawa taught?

In *The Book of Judgment* (G.O.M.F., 1980) he wrote:

> Man is a radio receiver and the infinite is the transmitter. This receiver works with millions and billions of vacuum microtubes. It is here that individual differences originate. The quality of these tubes depends upon their material and also upon the quality of the technique of their manufacture. The material is the food, and the technique is the selection and preparation of food and the manner in which it is consumed.
>
> That is why one can think of and understand the infinite and all that lies in it. That is why we can have infinitely numerous memories. That is why we can understand each other; our infinite brain is unique, yet common to the whole of humanity. That is why one can learn any language. That is why one perceives things that do not live within our sight but thousands of miles away, whether we are asleep or awake. And one can see what will happen in the future if his thinking is infinite, omnipresent, omnipotent, and omniscient.
>
> Herein lies the possibility of miracles. Memory, or heart, or the head that thinks and judges does not dwell in this little box called head; on the contrary, we are in the infinite which is called Head.

Also in *The Book of Judgment*, Ohsawa wrote on the origin of man: vegetal, element, pre-atomic, energy, yin-yang polarity, and finally oneness. "We now come to the conclusion that yin and yang are the left and right hands of the infinite – creator, destroyer, and reproducer of everything that exists." He called this yin and yang alternating concept of the world 'the order of the universe', and symbolized it by a logarithmic spiral. However, he didn't explain here where spirit or mind fit into this spiral. He explained it in another book, first published in 1940, called *The Order of the Universe*, never translated into English. A rough translation of part of it follows:

> Let us clarify spirit. First of all, spirit has no weight, size, time, life-length, and cannot be sensed by our sensory organs. It never ages. My spirit has always been the same, since childhood. Spirit has no physical power. Spirit cannot lift even one pound of stone. I am forty-nine years old now; my knowledge has increased but my spirit is the same as when I was seventeen or eighteen.
>
> Then where is the spirit? Some believe it is in the brain, some believe it is in the heart. However, nobody has found the spirit by autopsy.
>
> In order to locate the spirit, there is one key – thinking. Thinking is a function of spirit. Even though we don't know how our body is made, it is clear to us that we are able to think. What happens to this thinking ability when we are sleeping? Does it disappear? No. We have thinking ability even when we are sleeping. However, it appears in a different form. We call it a 'dream'.
>
> There are two kinds of dreams. One is unreasonable, unrealistic – the so-called 'dreamy' dream. Another is the true dream, by which one can see what is happening a thousand miles away, or see scenery one will encounter later. I often experienced such dreams after starting the macrobiotic diet, and confirmed thousands of people who have also experienced such true dreams.
>
> In any case, dreaming and thinking are mysterious things. I had a dream when I was a child of being a novelist. When my mother died, I dreamed of finding a way to prevent mothers from dying and leaving their small children behind. I had a dream to go to France and learn French. All my dreams have been miraculously realized. I don't know whether my life is a dream or the dream is my life.

Dreams have several distinct characteristics. First of all, a dream has no limit. We can dream anything, anytime, anywhere. Secondly, there is no physical pain or suffering. The world of dreaming is infinite. These characteristics are the same as those of the spiritual world. Therefore, 'dream' and 'spirit' are the same. When we are dreaming we are in an infinite and free world; by the same token, we are free and eternal when we are in the spiritual world.

The world of spirit is infinite and free, with no worry and with equality to all. This world could be called infinity, God, the universe, or the absolute world. The infinite world produced the finite, relative, yin and yang world. This creation happened not only billions of years ago but is happening now. In fact, this spirit or God is the creator of our world, our civilizations – the materialistic, unfree, and ephemeral world.

There are many books which teach this, such as the *Maka Hannya Hara Mitta Shin Gyo*, the *Tao Te Ching*, *The I Ching, The Upanishads*, the *Holy Bible*, etc. However, scholars have distorted the real meaning and modern people have lost the true meaning of spirit, thinking, and God's relation to this relative world. Due to this distortion this world is full of unhappiness, fighting, and disagreement. In order to clarify the understanding of spirit (world of thinking or infinity), I wrote this book and the diagram of the spiral. One who is suffering from unhappiness, please contemplate on my spiralic diagram of the order of the universe. There you will find the way to happiness.

Ohsawa's unique spiralic diagram appears on page 330 of this book.

Understanding Sickness

Modern medicine and laypeople alike misunderstand the cause of sickness.

When I visited Japan with sixteen American friends in May of this year, I met the famous Dr. Akizuki at his St. Francis Hospital in Nagasaki. He had saved his co-workers and patients from the inevitable radiation diseases that would have ensued after the World War II bombing by providing macrobiotic meals. He gave us a talk to express his criticism of Western medicine.

He said, "Western medicine is making the mistake of confusing the cause and effect of sickness. What Western medicine thinks is the cause of sickness is not the cause but actually the effect, or result of the cause. They are not treating the cause but the result – the mere symptom of sickness. Therefore, the treatments given by modern medicine are not curing disease, but merely keeping the symptoms from showing, thereby worsening the patient's condition."

This clearly points out the shortcomings of modern medicine. I have never before heard such a clear, accurate critique on Western medicine from a medical doctor. I was surprised and happy to hear such clear statements concerning modern medicine. I agree with his opinion without reservation, that what modern medicine thinks is the cause of sickness is not the cause at all but merely the symptom, or the effect of the cause.

For example, considering that pain is the cause of sickness, modern medicine tries to eliminate it by any means, never stopping to think what is the root cause of the pain. For instance, they see that swelling causes pain, so they try to reduce swelling without tracing the disease process back to what is causing the swelling. Since pain is not the cause of sickness, the elimination of the pain does not cure us; it just makes us think so. This is a false cure – really no cure at all, so sooner or later the pain and sickness come back again. Then patients are given painkillers and again think themselves cured when the pain stops. The sickness comes back again and again, but each time it's deeper rooted.

Modern medicine operates when breast cancer is found. Four to five years later the same patients are sick again, usually finding that their cancer has moved deeper into the body – very often to the lymphatic system or brain. At this time the sickness has scattered and cannot be operated on, so the doctors prescribe radiation or chemotherapy. With luck, the patient may live four or five more years. However, next time the cancer starts to be active there is very little left in the way of possible treatment.

In October of 1982 seven young people died by taking the pain-killing drug called Tylenol, which sells over the counter at drug stores all over the country. The deaths shocked the nation and led people to great fear and uncertainty. Since then nine months have passed but neither the criminals nor the cause have yet been found. Why did the Tylenol case happen? In my opinion, the drug-dependent mentality in this country was the real cause. If someone has a headache he buys a bottle of pills at one of the many convenient drugstores 'just around the corner' for an instant cure. Americans spent about $1 billion for cough and cold preparations, and $1.2 billion for internal analgesics in 1979 – this spending is going up every year.

This habit is the result of thinking that a headache is the cause of the sickness, whatever it may be; or just sentimental and egoistic thinking that "something has caused me pain and it should be stopped immediately by any means." This attitude has been cultivated by the medical profession in their view that the cause of most disease, infectious and otherwise, is germs (bacteria or viruses). Therefore, when people have pain or some kind of sickness, they think they have germs which are inflicting this pain and suffering on them and therefore feel justified in using any and all means to immediately wipe out the 'invaders'.

Here again is another confusion of cause and effect. Germs, whether bacteria or viruses, are not the cause of pain and sickness, even tuberculosis, but the effect of a weak condition which allows the germs access to the body. And even so, many people carry tuberculosis germs but only some will have an outbreak of the disease. What is the difference between those people who are affected by germs and those who are not? The difference lies in their physical constitution, diet, environment, stress, and mental attitude – which all determine their present condition.

Physical constitution is formed mainly during the fetal period from the mother's diet, which is most influenced by her diet, living environment, and the emotional stresses in her life at that time.

A woman living in a cold (yin) climate will probably eat much animal and other yang foods during her pregnancy, so her baby will tend to have a husky physical body and a more aggressive character. Someone born in a warmer climate, however, whose mother probably ate more fruits and yin foods during pregnancy, will tend to acquire a less physical, more fragile body and a less outward personality.

Constitution, environment, and stress in our lives greatly affect our health and happiness; however, our health and happiness are not necessarily destined by these factors. We can make ourselves healthy and happy even though we were born with a weak constitution, live in a poor environment, and endure much stress. In fact, many great men grow up under these conditions. Strength of character is developed by having to overcome negative influences in our lives.

In other words, the most important factors contributing to health and happiness, or a normal healthy condition, are one's current diet and mental attitude – coupled with the understanding that the symptoms of an illness are only the signs of an unbalanced condition. If you balance your condition you can overcome any obstacles to health and happiness.

How can diet help determine our sickness or health?

According to Dr. K. Morishita, in our body digested food (which is organic matter) transforms itself into the simplest life – a red blood cell; this simple life then transforms into a higher stage of life – a body cell (*Hidden Truth of Cancer*, G.O.M.F., 1976). Dr. K. Chishima voices this same opinion in his Japanese book, *K. Chishima's Work #9*. In modern physiology, however, the abovementioned theory is not accepted. It considers that foods give energy, protein, fats, vitamins, and minerals to cells, but that there is no direct relation with blood formation. Modern medicine believes that blood is formed in the bone marrow. This belief is based on an experiment performed in 1952 in which four physiologists, Drs. Donn, Cunningham, Sabin, and Jordan, performed a two-week starvation experiment using chickens and doves. From their results they concluded that all red blood cells are produced from bone marrow.

However, Dr. Morishita argues differently. He says, "When fasting, the cells of the bone marrow, adipose tissue, muscular tissue, liver, etc., transform back to red blood cells in that order, beginning with the bone marrow. Therefore, what the four physiologists witnessed was not normal blood production because the animals were not being fed during the experiment. Normal physiological blood production is done by the intestine. When fasting, however, and also in case of stomach illness and intestinal diarrhea, the intestine halts its production of red blood cells and the body cells start reverse transformation to red blood cells."

According to Chishima and Morishita, food not only changes to red blood cells but red blood cells then change to soma, or tissue, cells. Dr. Morishita says, "Modern medicine distinguishes between the red blood cell and the tissue cell. In reality, however, they are related to each other and can be transformed in both directions. When a person is healthy the red blood cells change to body cells; when one is sick the reverse will happen."

Macrobiotics agrees with this opinion and says food transforms to body cells. Ohsawa said that one-tenth of the body's blood cells die every day. Therefore, in about ten days we totally renew our blood. (From this thought came the idea of the ten-day rice diet.) He said, further, that body cells, which have an average life span of seven years, are continually dying and being replaced. Therefore, if we change our diet, we will be able to change the quality of all of our body cells in about seven years.

Thus macrobiotics believes that food first changes to red blood cells, which then transform into body cells. The most basic cause of sickness is a weak blood condition from poor quality food. Sickness develops in a specific order: from food – to blood – to cells.

Stages of Sickness

There are seven main stages of sickness. The first stage of sickness is fatigue which is the result of overeating, too much sugary food, and no orderliness in living conditions.

The second stage of sickness is pain, which is the result of poor blood circulation; not getting enough oxygen supply to the body cells because of broken and blocked capillaries. One of the most direct indications of this is chest pain, which occurs when coronary heart capillaries are blocked by fat and blood cannot reach the heart tissue cells in adequate supply. Whenever cells do not get enough oxygen we feel pain as a warning signal.

The third stage of sickness is infectious disease. This is the result of yin quality or acidic body fluid due to the overeating of sugar, honey, sweeteners, fruits, spices, alcohol, drugs, refined foods, and processed foods. Herpes and AIDS fall in this stage of sickness. Body cells are normally surrounded by intercellular fluids which are very much like ocean water – always alkaline and a little bit salty. If this fluid is sweet (yin) or too acidic, cells which are living in this internal ocean will start decomposing due to bacterial growth. This is infectious disease.

The fourth stage of sickness is weakness of the autonomic nervous system, which controls hormone secretions and organ function. This is caused by a progressive worsening of the first three stages and is also caused by accidents which deform the spine, inhibiting nerve impulses to the organs. Continuing to eat sugary foods, animal foods, and fatty foods causes the body fluid to turn acidic, slowing down nerve cell function and then hormone secretion. When hormonal secretion is abnormal, the work of all organs is disturbed. Thus thyroid, pancreas (insulin secretion), and kidney/adrenal cortex (cortical hormone secretion) problems begin.

The fifth stage of sickness is disease of the cells and organs – cancer. Our body fluid must be alkaline, normally pH 7.4. This is accurately maintained by the normal functions of our organs, especially the kidneys which filter out acids. However, when the kidneys become weak, the body fluid starts becoming acidic. If the body fluid reaches pH 6.9, cells die. However, between pH 6.9 and pH 7.0 the cells, instead of dying, start to change their gene structure so that they can survive an acidic condition, or they produce new cells which are adapted to such an environment. This is the start of malignant or cancer cells.

The first cause of this acidity is synthetic chemicals in foods such as flavorings, preservatives, dyes, conditioners, etc. Some of them are known to be carcinogenic, but even so-called 'safe' chemicals can be highly dangerous if combined with other 'safe' chemicals. Cancer patients especially must avoid all chemicalized foods.

The next acid-forming food is fat. Eating high fat food is taking the expressway to cancer, as fat metabolism produces large amounts of acid wastes, and almost all cancer patients have eaten a lot of animal foods and other foods rich in fats.

The third acid-forming food is sugar and foods with sugar added. Sugar destroys red blood cells, depletes oxygen and vitamins, causes anemia, and increases carbon dioxide (a by-product of its metabolism), thus causing an acidic condition.

Fruits are not acid-forming foods, but we do not recommend them for cancer patients because they contain so much fruit sugar, which makes the blood yin – weakening the immune system. Fruit sugar also readily changes to fat, which then clogs the blood vessels, impairing circulation.

The sixth stage of sickness is a psychological one. One who complains a lot belongs in this group (emotional, schizophrenic, neurasthenic, etc.). It is caused by all the physical causes mentioned above, and/or family education and upbringing.

The seventh stage of sickness is spiritual. This is the state of mind which has no gratitude, no appreciation, and no faith in the order of the universe.

This seven-stage cycle can be viewed in reverse, originating at the seventh (spiritual) level and then carrying over into the physical.

Living is a wonderful thing. It is especially a miracle to live in this money-oriented, greed-controlled society. When we do not appreciate our life, that is the very deepest sickness of all.

People come to our study house and, just by observing a balanced diet, stop pains which have lasted many years. Some of them still do not appreciate what this good food has done for them, and as soon as the pain goes away they start eating badly again. This mentality is sickness of the seventh stage.

Many people cure so-called incurable diseases by observing a macrobiotic diet. However, few of them really appreciate what they learn. Even fewer give others what they have learned. Those people again become sick sooner or later. After many years of macrobiotic teaching, I have learned that a person who appreciates and has gratitude can cure any sickness, even cancer.

Give Me Time

Due to the scientific experiments done by O. Frank of Germany and E.H. Storing of England it is clear that the heart muscle can beat by itself. They kept a dog's heart active after separating it from all nerves and bodily systems. In *The Human Organism* (Basic Books, Inc., 1966), David F. Horrobin wrote, "We do not have to stimulate the nerves to the heart or the heart muscle artificially in order to make it contract; in this respect it is very different from ordinary muscles. If care is taken to keep the muscle in good condition, even isolated strips of heart will continue to beat. All heart muscle can, under the right conditions, beat rhythmically by itself."

Alexis Carrel kept pieces of a chicken's heart alive and beating for twenty-eight years after extracting it by keeping it in a saline (salt) solution, which he changed daily.

Why does the heart pulsate?

Using Oriental philosophy this can be answered very easily. Yang is a contracting force and yin is an expanding force. If there is a yang force in the heart, the heart contracts. If there is a yin force outside the heart, the heart expands. The result is the pulsation of the heart.

What is the internal yang force of the heart? It is that heart muscles contain large amounts of the element sodium (relative to potassium). What is the yin force outside the heart? It is the large amounts of potassium (relative to sodium) in the intercellular fluid and space outside the heart.

Most macrobiotic students know that potassium is more yin than sodium, and that therefore sodium is more yang than potassium. We know that vegetables are rich in potassium, therefore vegetal foods are more yin. Conversely, animal tissue is rich in sodium, therefore animal foods have a more yang quality. However, most are not aware that we are living between the two greatest forces of yin and yang. That is to say, space (yin) and gravitation (yang). Without these two forces nothing on the earth could exist. Without space's expansive force (yin) everything would shrink to nothing, and without gravitation's contractive force (yang) everything would expand endlessly.

These two forces are the cause of the ocean waves which are producing billions and billions of watts of energy every second all over the world. Ocean waves pulsate for the same reason as a chicken's heart.

When I came to America in September of 1952, I rode a Swedish cargo boat from Yokohama to San Francisco via the northern Pacific Ocean, passing by the shore of Alaska. It was typhoon season so the ocean was extremely rough. A typhoon passed by and the boat pitched and rolled badly. One of the sailors got washed out on the deck and was injured. The boat returned at once to Yokohama where the injured boy was hospitalized and we set off again.

There were eight passengers. Six of them were students going to study in American universities and two were Americans who had been studying in Japan and were on their way home. All of these passengers got seasick at various times and couldn't come to the dining room at meal time. I was the only one who never missed a meal. I was not seasick at all although the boat would go up and down twenty to thirty feet at a time. Why was I able to be free from seasickness? Because I was always on the deck watching the wave movement. The wave motion fascinated me. I wondered what is the cause of wave motion which does not relate to tides. Wave height seemed to me to be related to weather: when it was colder the waves were higher. But it did not seem to be directly related to the wind as some scientists claim, because even when we had no wind there were still large waves; but when the wind blew in colder air, the waves did get higher. Also the waves were higher when we were way out from shore, out in the open seas. From this experience I concluded that the cause of waves is as follows:

Ocean water with salt is yang and is receiving the gravitational downward pull, which is also yang, all the time. However, the space above the water is very yin. It is more yin out over open water, such as the Pacific Ocean, and is less yin near islands or continents. It is more yin when the weather is colder (rainy, windy, cloudy, snowy, etc.). Space, being yin, attracts the yang water below. Ocean water is thus pulled up. However, movement stops when this yin upward motion is balanced by yang gravitational power, which pulls the ocean water back downward again.

Since the ocean's salt concentration and gravitational pulling power at sea level is about the same all over the earth, the height of waves depends more on how yin the space above is. This is the reason that when the weather in an area is colder the waves there are higher, as they are when farther from the shore.

Not only is ocean water receiving the two forces of space's pulling power and gravitational downward power, but the whole earth and everything on it are also influenced by these powers; everything is influenced by space (yin) and gravitation (yang) all the time. This brings us to another mysterious factor that exists in the universe – time. Time is more yang than space and more yin than gravitation.

Space and time have similar characteristics. Both can be cut smaller and smaller endlessly and enlarged endlessly; they both shrink and expand infinitely. However, they are opposites in their overall influence. Space gives yin-power and time gives yang-power. Living in a large house or land such as America makes one more yin, whereas decreasing space by living in a small house or country such as Japan makes one more yang. In America there seems to be more time as well as space, whereas in Japan there seems to be less of both.

But time has no duration. Time is instant – it exists only at the present. Past and future exist in our brain as memory or thought but not in reality. Therefore, time can be considered yang. However, people use the word 'time' as a duration. In this case, time is yin and has a meaning similar to space. For example, "give me more time" or "I have more time" have the connotation of relaxation. Therefore, in these cases, time is used as yin, such as space.

The Bible says in Matthew 17:20 that if you have faith as a grain of mustard seed, you can say to a mountain to move, and the mountain will move, and nothing will be impossible. This is difficult to accept as a rational statement rather than a rhetorical one. However, we can understand why this is possible when we apply infinite time (absolute yin) to the saying.

Everything changes. What are now mountains were under the ocean at one time or several times in the history of the universe. Even the highest mountain which is elevated above the earth will sometime again be under the water. This is possible when we give infinite time. This time is not an instant but an infinitely long duration. During infinite time, a mountain will move.

Infinite time makes everything possible. This is called faith. In other words, faith – which is absolute yin, or infinity – changes yang time to yin time. Therefore, anything can happen – even impossible things such as making mountains move.

An Aid to AIDS

Americans are facing diseases today for which cures, or even causes, have not been found – even with the technologically advanced medical research of today. They are cancer, herpes, and AIDS. Since no cures are even remotely in sight and these diseases are spreading like epidemics, they are directly influencing many facets in the lives and lifestyles of the American public. Many cancer patients are now radically changing their diets, even to macrobiotics, which is quite a change from mainstream eating patterns. Herpes and AIDS are both having a profound effect on sexual relationships.

"The truth about life in the United States in the 1980s," says Dr. Kevin Murphy of Dallas, one of the nation's leading herpes researchers, "is that if you are going to have sex, you are going to have to take the risk of getting herpes." (*Time*, August 2, 1982.)

The article continues:

> An estimated 20 million Americans (about 10% of the population) now have genital herpes, with as many as half a million new cases expected this year, according to the Center for Disease Control in Atlanta. These remarkable numbers are altering sexual rites in America, changing courtship patterns.
>
> Many 'swingers' have dropped out because of herpes. Wives now give husbands smiling lectures on the

ravages of disease to keep them faithful. Many middle-aged men refuse to date women under 30 in the belief that younger people are more likely to have herpes. Some marriages, and many relationships, end in discord and the lingering suspicion caused by herpes.

For all the distress it has brought, the troublesome little bug may inadvertently be ushering in a period in which sex is linked more firmly to commitment and trust.

Now another serious disease is changing American life – AIDS. This is becoming epidemic among homosexuals, and is another warning that one is violating the universal order.

In ancient China there was a beautiful lady of the court named Daki. The lord loved her so much that he gave her everything she asked for, even the life of the most royal of his chamberlains. Since she was a very egoistic lady, she didn't like the royal samurai who would give their honest opinions to the lord. She asked him to fire or kill such samurai, and he followed her wishes. As the result, his country became so weak that an enemy then destroyed it easily. Therefore, in China or in Japan, such beautiful but egoistic women are called 'Kei Koku' – one who destroys country or men.

The Kei Koku of twentieth century America are not women but men. Homosexuals make men the victims of AIDS.

In January 1981, a thirty-one year old male model arrived at the emergency room of UCLA Medical Center with a fungal infection in his throat so severe that it almost completely blocked his esophagus. This symptom showed that his immune system was very weak. Two weeks later, he developed a lung inflammation which is seen only in the case of lung cancer.

A few months later, two more patients with similar lung inflammation showed up. Dr. M.S. Gottlieb was puzzled because of the unusual symptoms and the fact that they were all homosexuals. About the same time, Dr. A. Friedman-Kien of New York University noted that several of his homosexual patients had the same weakened immune systems and Kaposi's sarcoma, a rare cancer of the skin usually seen only in older men. Dr. Friedman-Kien called a friend at the University of California Medical Center in San Francisco and found there were two homosexual cases of Kaposi's sarcoma there.

AIDS victims had increased to 1,641 by July 1983 and about 165 new victims are now added every month; the numbers are increasing.

"AIDS attacks its victims by knocking out the immune system," wrote *Time* on July 4, 1983, "thus leaving them defenseless against a host of 'opportunistic' infections. A rare form of cancer or pneumonia becomes a deadly invader, but so does fungus or a common virus. Thus far, there is no cure for AIDS and its source remains unknown." These various microorganisms, including a variety of fungi, are constantly present at various sites in the body – notably the mucous membranes. However, a healthy immune system keeps their growth in check. A normal immune system has twice as many helper T-cells, which stimulate the making of antibodies, than suppressor T-cells, which suppress antibody production. In AIDS victims, this ratio is reversed. They are therefore easily affected by infections, and the growth of unfriendly micro-organisms becomes out of control.

These points remind me of the life of salmon. When the salmon swim upriver to spawn, females lay eggs on the river bed and a following male deposits sperm over the eggs. After all eggs and sperm are spent, both the male and female are left extremely yin and lose their immune power. The result of this weakening is the growth of fungus all over their bodies, and within a short time they completely decompose. AIDS victims are experiencing similar circumstances, partially as a result of having intercourse more frequently than their condition allows. As reported by *Time*, "The average AIDS victim has had 60 different sexual partners in the past 12 months." Having sex so frequently they lose a lot of sperm, which is a transformation of blood. In excess, this weakens the blood and tends to put them in an extremely yin condition, unless they are very yang to begin with. They lose the power of their immune system, which then allows fungi and other detrimental organisms to develop. The victims have depleted their yang energy.

However, the loss of too much sperm is not the only cause. Receiving sperm, such as in the case of a passive partner, can also cause AIDS. The reason for this is simple. Sperm is extremely yin; it makes an egg conceive. The egg then grows three billion times in just nine months. This ability to cause expansion illustrates sperm's very yin quality. Homosexual passive partners receive this yin sperm in the intestine where it is absorbed directly into the bloodstream, making the blood very yin. This again causes one to lose the power of the immune system.

Prevention of AIDS is easier than a cure. One must keep the blood quality strong through proper diet and lifestyle, and regulate sexual relations according to one's condition.

Happy New Year 1984

1984 is a Year of the Mouse according to the Japanese folk calendar. The mouse is the symbolic character of grain-eaters and hard laborers; mice are seen as the unappreciated supporters of the economy in that they have an unusually keen sensitivity for knowing when calamity will strike. The Japanese have observed that the entire mouse population of a town will disappear just days before a major earthquake or flood hits. Many have relied on this ability in that land of severe natural catastrophes. This hints that the year 1984 is not to be a year of fame and outward prosperity, but should be spent preparing for more prosperous times in the future.

According to the Chinese calendar, 1984 is the year of *Ne*. This is the state of planting where the seeds have been sown and are accumulating the energy needed for germination. During this time, the plants spend their time immersed in the soil. Their activities are not known or outwardly seen from above, but they are nonetheless preparing for their coming appearance.

These two views of 1984 have inspired the following advice to macrobiotic leaders. In the last couple of years macrobiotics has been highly publicized on television and in magazines. As a result, requests for macrobiotic classes, consultations, and books have mushroomed, increasing probably five times in this short period.

This widespread popularity (a yin quality) coupled with reports of irresponsible consultations has drawn the attention (a yang quality) of the medical community. In February of 1984 hearings will be conducted by a Senate Subcommittee on Long Term Health Care for the Aged. Macrobiotics has been lumped in with quack schemes that take advantage of the elderly through mail order rip-offs, etc. Medical authorities are not happy with any unorthodox method, especially if it is not yet highly documented as a success. Of course, a cautious attitude regarding treatments is warranted; there are many making lots of money without delivering real benefits in macrobiotics too.

Macrobiotic people who are giving consultations should be very careful in not making over-enthusiastic promises regarding treatments. Of course macrobiotics is effective but not everyone can benefit. My advice is that consultations should be limited to dietary recommendations. Time should be devoted primarily to the teaching of macrobiotics rather than the treatment of sickness.

If macrobiotic leaders are too interested in becoming rich and famous, 1984 may well see macrobiotics pushed underground, not unlike the germination period experienced in the 1960s. We should proceed carefully – we are not yet strong enough to be unscathed by opposition. If we advance too quickly, a strong attack could hurt our cause. This would be all right in that we would inevitably gather strength for a new appearance, but I think the better way may be to pace ourselves and be content with smooth progress towards our goals until we get strong and established enough that we can quell a strong assault and use it to our benefit. As the mouse we should be the little seen, and probably not very appreciated, contributors to society in 1984.

Macrobiotic Leadership

Who is a leader? What is a leader? Who wants to be a leader in the future? You must know what is the quality of a leader. I asked this of George Ohsawa twenty years ago; he was my current age then in New York City. Now I am his age here. Ohsawa said, "I will wait ten years. Then you and Michio take over my position." He left exactly ten years later. So now Michio and I are looking for a leader to take over the movement.

If you have too many qualifications, you cannot do it. It's better to only have a few.

The first condition of leadership is trustworthiness. In 1961 the New York macrobiotic group organized the Second Macrobiotic Summer Camp at Watsboro, New York, inviting George Ohsawa from France as the sole lecturer.

One day at the camp during a rare resting time, he was sitting comfortably outside the building. I was with him, talking generally about the macrobiotic situation in New York (the only macrobiotic activity in the United States at that time). For one moment he stopped talking and then started again with the most important words that I have heard in my life.

"Macrobiotics in America will be all right. It will survive in America."

"Why do you say that?" I asked.

He answered me simply, "Because people trust Michio and you."

What glory, joy, and honor I felt. I said no words. I just felt a great honor because he was counting on me for the future of macrobiotics in America.

Since then I have tried to be a man who could be trusted by family, friends, and people. I do not think I gained people's trust 100 percent; however, I tried all the time. If I have become a leader in the American macrobiotic movement, one reason must be that I have gained some trust from people. Therefore, my first condition of leadership is 'to be trusted by all'. You must do what you promise. You have to be honest. For instance, you make a commitment at a meeting – that is easy. But the hard thing comes after, when you have to follow up. Otherwise this meeting is a waste of time; better to go to the park and play baseball.

The next qualification of a leader is respect. You have to respect all people, and then you will have the respect of others. If you respect ten people, you are the leader of ten; if you respect one hundred people, you are the leader of one hundred; if you respect one thousand, you are the leader of one thousand, and so on. If your communication is without respect, it's a dead end – it gets clogged up, like the body does from a high-cholesterol diet.

The next condition of leadership is 'no exclusivity'. Why is 'no exclusivity' the condition of a leader, and what is it?

'No exclusivity' is a state of mind with which one understands and lives Oneness or Totality. A leader must unite a group of people as one. Therefore, he must understand, as well as live with, 'no exclusivity'.

Exclusivity is one of the natural manifestations of ego. As long as we have an ego, we live with some exclusivity. Therefore, there are always wars, hatred, separation, and antagonism in all human life.

It is almost impossible to attain 'no exclusivity' in our lives. Exclusivity is biological; 'no exclusivity' is spiritual. 'No exclusivity' exists only in the spiritual world, or Supreme Consciousness. One who attains this Supreme Consciousness is the true leader.

Today exclusivity is the life principle; societies, nations, families, and individuals are governed by exclusivity. Immigration law is exclusive. Modern medicine is based on it, because orthodox medicine excludes other methods of medicine and treatment. All religions exclude each other. To be successful in industry or business today, it's inevitable to be exclusive. Now even families are breaking their unity, due to their members' exclusivity.

Ohsawa's medicine was to live with no exclusivity – to accept even sickness, bacteria, pain, and tumors. Ohsawa's medicine is not to eliminate bacteria, viruses, or tumors, but to make them your friends your benefactors

He used to say, "I never met a man I didn't like." Bahai's leader said, "Love your enemies." Christ said, "Give your left cheek if someone hits your right cheek." This is 'no exclusivity', and love.

I have not reached such a state of mind. Therefore, I am not a leader. However, I am trying to reach this state so that I can love all people.

Since 99 percent of people are exclusive, the one who has no exclusivity will be a true leader. There have been few such leaders in human history. Today, wars and antagonism cover the face of the earth. The cause of this lies in the fact that there is no real leader in today's world society, whether political or spiritual.

The fourth condition the leader must satisfy is that he must have judgment which will make him happy and healthy. If he can't make himself happy and healthy, he is not a qualified leader. One's happiness and health depend on judgment. Such good judgment is the fourth condition of leadership.

In order to be a macrobiotic leader, however, being able to be happy and healthy is not enough. One must be able to make one's family, friends, and society happy and healthy as well.

In today's society, people select their leaders from candidates who claim to be able to make people happy, even though they are not happy themselves since they are not healthy. There is no real way of knowing their true value, so voters' judgments mostly depend on mass media advertisements which are paid for by the candidates or their supporters. When societies are controlled by such leaders, it is obvious that the future will not be so happy or healthy.

The fifth condition of the macrobiotic leader is having extreme humbleness, so that he can never be arrogant or proud of his ability or success.

When I was a college student, I attended a lecture entitled World Concept Seminar given by four distinguished scholars. The first one was Chikao Fujisawa, a Shintoist who gave a lecture on Japanese religion or Shinto. The second lecturer was Shumei Ohkawa, a famous authority on German history who was the theoretical organizer of the Japanese military government. The third was a religious teacher named Shuzo Takado. The last one was George Ohsawa.

I was impressed most by Ohsawa's talk in which he discussed the yin and yang concept as the basis of an understanding of East and West. Next, I was most impressed by the talk of Mr. Takado, who said, "I look at people with great admiration because I feel they are more honest, innocent, and human than I am." I still remember that night, over forty years ago. Ohsawa gave me an intellectual shock; Takado gave me a spiritual shock.

Ohsawa said he never met a man he didn't like. Mr. Takado said he never met a man who is not greater than he although he was a great scholar, writer, and leader of the spiritual movement in Japan. What a humble man he was. Since then I have been thinking that the fifth condition of leadership is the humility of Shuzo Takado.

Having such humbleness and no exclusivity, such a person will receive the help of many people who will help him without his asking. Such a person is a real macrobiotic leader.

Always open yourself up. When we moved from New York to Chico we had several families, thirty-six people; we found out we were an exclusive group of people – for instance, looking after only our own children and not each others'. If you want to influence the world, you have to be inclusive of everyone in the world.

And if you want world peace, you have to start with your neighbors. 'One peaceful world' must begin with many happy communities.

April 1984

Macrobiotics and Medicine: A Balance

We asked our Foundation members to write to congressmen about our view of macrobiotics, so that the House of Representatives' Subcommittee on Health and Long Term Care would receive opinions different from those they may otherwise hear. Since then, several of our members responded and wrote to their congressmen, most of whom answered with favorable words.

Due to those responses, I think I have found the key point which may or may not make the macrobiotic movement into another Beth Ann Simon case. [She was a drug addict who died in the sixties while following a highly restricted diet.] That is to say, in a few words: an exclusive and fanatical attitude to macrobiotics, and practicing medicine without a license, will be the key factors that determine whether macrobiotic practice will continue in this country.

In consultations, it is hard to draw a line defining what is meant by practicing medicine. Of course, if all the persons seen by macrobiotic consultants cured their sicknesses and had better health, then probably no problems would arise. However, in reality, some of them will not get better; some of them will die. In such cases, how will macrobiotic consultants, or the macrobiotic movement, become the target of condemnation for practicing medicine?

In my opinion, it is the exclusive and fanatical attitude that

254

may be shown toward sick persons. In *Anatomy of an Illness* (W. W. Norton and Co., Inc., 1979), Norman Cousins stresses the importance of diet but he also recommends that the wholistic health movement as well as the medical profession should exercise good judgment:

> It is a serious error to suppose . . . that medication can accomplish a desired purpose despite everything else that is taken into the human body, or that the right foods cannot be used effectively to fight disease, whether in combination with medication or without it. . . . It is reasonable to expect the doctor to accord nutrition a high place in the understanding and treatment of illness. It is equally reasonable to expect him to listen to his patient's own developed interest in the subject, even though the doctor may see logical and factual gaps in the patient's articulation.
>
> It is unreasonable, however, to expect a physician to believe that the right foods, however essential, are all that is required to cure any disease. What is needed here – as it is in all matters – is a sense of balance, that neither attempts to dismiss vitamins out of hand, nor regards them as the only key to good health. Such a balance is possible, given attitudes of reasonableness, by both physician and patient. The wholistic health movement can discover its greatest effectiveness by seeking such a balance.

Since Ohsawa condemned symptomatic modern medicine as ineffective and recommended diet for curing almost any sickness without reservation, someone who has the common sense mentioned by Cousins will naturally think macrobiotics is exclusive, fanatical, and a dangerous healing method.

Someone who has experienced the miraculous power of the macrobiotic diet will not wonder at Ohsawa's claim; however, someone who never experienced that curing power will think that the diet is a fake and that the followers are crazy.

As long as the macrobiotic movement is small, nobody cares

what it claims. However, when the macrobiotic movement becomes big and famous, the medical profession starts to be concerned about Ohsawa's claims ("No illness is more simple to cure than cancer"). Ohsawa made such claims in order to draw the attention of the public and also to emphasize the effectiveness of the diet. However, this is true only for a person who could understand very well and would observe the macrobiotic diet wisely. Ohsawa's claim is idealistic but reality is different. Ohsawa knew this, but he wanted to be an idealist.

Now the American congress is investigating the macrobiotic approach. They should understand that what is claimed in *Zen Macrobiotics* is idealism and not reality; that what macrobiotic students are aiming at is a world of perfect health, longevity, and world peace, where food is the medicine. At this time of an 'unhealthy-civilized' society, macrobiotic teachers and followers should be willing to cooperate with medical authorities and to give all their knowledge of macrobiotic medicine to the doctors to help suffering people, even those who have been given up by doctors.

Norman Cousins thinks we need a balance between conventional medicine and the macrobiotic diet. I am ready if any medical doctor wants my advice for his patients. If this congressional investigation can ignite cooperation between conventional medicine and macrobiotics, the benefit to the sick as well as the healthy will be great.

That will be the real macrobiotic way of thinking, because it makes your enemy your friend, and changes bad luck to good luck.

How Change Changes

Sick people often make a mistake in their expectations of recovery. When they start the macrobiotic diet many of them expect a certain amount of improvement immediately, and for this to continue every day. However, in actuality this is not usually the case.

In most cases the improvement appears only after several days of the diet – probably seven to ten days or longer. Then, for another while no change appears. When people start doubting the diet, a second improvement often appears. A third improvement may appear after even a longer interval.

In short, these changes follow a stepped and not a linear pattern.

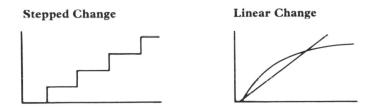

Stepped Change   **Linear Change**

In the stepped pattern there are no changes for a time, and then there is a sudden change. In the linear pattern, some changes happen every day in a certain proportion; a graph will be closer to a straight line or curve, but not the zigzag line of a stepped change.

The effect of a macrobiotic diet on sickness begins with a change of blood quality, which will happen a little each day. However, this change of blood quality has very little obvious influence on the condition of cells and on the sick organs and muscles, or the accumulation of cells. Therefore, the immediate influence of the diet is so small that we notice the changes not every day, but a while later. Understanding of this change is important, because if we understand it we will not be disappointed in our progress.

Another reason for the importance of this understanding is seen when we are healthy. Then, each time we binge, symptoms may not appear unless we are very weak. So someone may think that it is okay to binge every day; then the bad diet changes blood quality, and then eventually cell quality, and finally organ dysfunction or pain results. These symptoms appear suddenly rather than as gradual changes. The tendency for the change to not appear for a certain number of days will be greater when the person is stronger, because a stronger person can hold more toxicity. Therefore, the stronger person tends to acquire worse sickness than the weaker.

One such case is cancer. In other words, the person who is stronger will have more chance to develop cancer than the weaker one.

Practicing the macrobiotic diet for a long time (more than about seven years) makes us very strong physically, even if we had been weak previously. Such a strong person can binge but no sickness may appear right away, or even for six months. Then symptoms of sickness can appear suddenly. At that time the sickness is so deep that recovery takes time, even following a strict diet. In such a case, some people may doubt the validity of a macrobiotic diet. Some may even quit it and take symptomatic medicine. Such a person usually ends up with severe sickness by worsening the condition each time he receives medication.

Another path for change is the spiralic way of change. There are two aspects of spiralic change. One is centrifugal and the other is centripetal.

Sickness starts at the center – the blood – and reaches all over the body. Therefore, the development of sickness is centrifugal. It is the same with curing; it starts at the center with the blood, and again reaches all over the body.

However, the speed pattern of both sickness and curing is slow at the beginning, becoming faster, thus forming a centripetal spiral.

The last pattern of change is a cyclic one. These changes are manifested in natural rhythmic cycles. Our daily activity, hunger, bowel movement, sugar metabolism, etc., are changing by daily or hourly cycles. Then there are the monthly cycles, like menstruation or ovulation.

Our heartbeat is governed by a one-second cycle, and we breathe with a four-second cycle. When we do heavy exercise these cycles become faster, but in any case they still change in cyclic rhythms. It seems to me that the movement of the heart relates to the rhythmic movement of the ocean wave. And sexual cycles are related to moon changes.

One of the most important effects of these cycles is the cycle of foods. Animals are more influenced by the moon cycle; thus, when we eat animal foods we come under more of a monthly influence, bringing about more abrupt emotional changes caused by animal-produced hormones. When we eat vegetal foods, we are influenced by their growth cycles (grains require almost a year to mature), resulting in calmer emotions.

The growth of plants change by the month too, as well as relating to the sun cycle. Then there must be cyclic changes that are influenced by Venus, Mercury, Mars, or other planets. Ancient people acknowledged the cyclic changes of the stars, and made calendars to show them.

The 18th Ohsawa Memorial

George Ohsawa scolded the students in his class severely when they were lazy, did not show initiative, were not making judgments by themselves, had no order in their thinking and doing, and, especially, when they made excuses. He severely scolded anyone who made excuses in order to pretend that he was not responsible for his situation. Many students were offended when they were scolded for their mistakes in front of other students – and their excuses brought more scoldings.

Many students would make excuses whenever they were accused of wrongdoings. Ohsawa never accepted excuses, even though they sounded reasonable. Sometimes students felt they were right. However, Ohsawa never allowed them to excuse themselves. In his school there were no excuses for being lazy, making mistakes, doing a sloppy job, not answering questions, or not writing reports.

In short, 'no excuse' was his education. Why did he so strongly insist that there is no excuse? The reason is simple. Excusing one's own responsibilities does not make one happy, but rather unhappier in the long run.

In modern society, people live on excuses. It seems that whoever makes the most excuses achieves the most success in their status, position, etc. Workers who make good excuses receive raises in salary. If someone admits his mistake without an excuse, he may lose his job. If someone doesn't make a good excuse for his crime, he may end up with a heavier penalty. Today's justice depends on how good or bad is the excuse.

Is Ohsawa's 'no excuse' education, then, obsolete? I don't think so. In my opinion, excuses work temporarily and in the short term. However good your excuse is, if you don't correct your mistakes or wrongdoings, people do not accept a second excuse. Therefore, an excuse is not the final solution but only symptomatic.

More importantly, someone who makes excuses all the time will lose credibility and trust. In other words, each time he makes excuses he is issuing counterfeit money.

Another reason why 'no excuse' is a good policy is that an excuse may be accepted by humans, but not by nature. A mistake in your diet may cause some sickness such as coughing, cold, pain, etc. Your wife accuses you of having drunk too much, and you blame your bad friend, etc. However, you cannot make that excuse for nature – that pain or sickness. Nature gives us the exact amount of punishment that corresponds to the size of the mistake we make. For this reason, Ohsawa never scolded macrobiotic students when they became sick. He didn't need to.

Summer 1984

A Trip to Mexico City

At the end of April, Cornellia and I went to Mexico City for a twelve-day lecture trip. We left at 4:30 in the morning. It was cool and we carried winter clothes in our baggage because people advised us that it would be cold at the high elevation of Mexico City.

I was very excited to visit Mexico City. Ever since twenty Mexicans came to our French Meadows Summer Camp nine years ago I had wanted to visit the country of the Aztec and Mayan civilizations.

My trip was very miserable at first; I had a headache for three days and then diarrhea for five days. However, it turned out to be a very enjoyable trip. I came back home with love for many Mexican macrobiotic friends. They like us so much that I felt as if they were my sons and daughters. Now, Mexico is no longer just another strange country located south of the United States. When I look at a map of Mexico, my mind vividly sees the macrobiotic center of Mexico City; the third floor room where I stayed for twelve days; the bakery which is located on the roof; the elderly lady who makes delicious macrobiotic cake and bread; Carola who owns the building (and gives cooking classes and lectures without salary to maintain the center); and the many volunteers who come to the center from early morning to late night – cleaning the kitchen, mopping the floor, cooking and baking, answering telephones, and selling macrobiotic foods – cheerfully and without being paid.

The center is like a blooming lily in the mud pond. People working there are like singing birds in the jungle. One step outside is the never-ending noise of Mexico City's streets, where you see nothing but mass-produced merchandise or poisoned foods. It is a miracle that such a macrobiotic organization exists in the center of a city that is three times more highly populated and polluted than Los Angeles. It is a miracle that a three-story building is owned and operated by one young lady who does not know business, but holds a Ph.D. in space-time mathematics.

Even though I stayed only twelve days, I saw several problems existing in Mexico:

1. One-third of the plants in the parks that we visited in Mexico City are dying. There are no sprinkler systems in the parks and the air is polluted. I had a headache for the first three days because of the bad air. You cannot see the sun in this city.

2. The banks are owned by the government. However, the government is not banking for the people but for themselves (I think). Therefore, banking in Mexico is terrible; for example, the loan interest rate is 60 percent. Nobody dares to borrow from the bank, except the gangsters. In my opinion, Mexico's financial situation is critical.

3. Many of the townspeople are low in social judgment. For example, I saw many drivers going through red traffic signals as long as there were no cars coming. In other words, people are not relying on the government's rules but on their own. Such a tendency may lead to political explosion.

4. The original Mexicans are becoming extinct. The present Mexicans are a mixture of Spanish or Caucasian and American Indian. Those who have adapted to Western civilization seem to be rich and have high status. Those who do not adapt, especially to the Spanish influence, seem very poor and have hatred for any white people, even though the Spanish culture has been well mixed into the Mexican culture. It seems

to me that the true Mexican culture now is overly influenced by Spanish culture. It is very difficult to distinguish the original. This is similar to the situation in Japan. It is very difficult to distinguish the Japanese people's own culture as opposed to that which has been influenced by China, India, and the West. All cultures are blending to form one culture in this highly developed technological civilization. Therefore, no such thing as 'pure culture' exists anymore.

Macrobiotic people in Mexico are an elite intelligentsia. They are the leaders of the Mexico that is coming, although they are too yin right now. However, they are very serious about learning macrobiotics. They are following the macrobiotic diet very seriously. These people are much more spiritual than the North American macrobiotic people that I know of, because they are more appreciative and grateful for the teaching of macrobiotics.

It is my opinion that these few Mexican macrobiotic people will lead not only Mexicans but also Americans in the future.

Thoughts on Marriage
From a talk at Vega

Some people are more happy married, some more happy alone. Marriage is very difficult; as one person you may have enough trouble, so as two people you may have even more. But I see that most people have four times the trouble – each one has double. Sometimes it feels like that, if you are not lucky. I see very few who have a happy marriage.

In my opinion, if you expect a happy marriage, then you will be disappointed, and it will end in divorce (that's why arranged marriages often work better). You have to make happiness – happiness doesn't come to you. It's never given, though many people expect it.

When we lived in New York, we were a very close community. I didn't meet many American macrobiotic people, but after moving to California we met more Americans. One man said to me, "My wife is so wonderful" . . . he admired her from top to bottom . . . then, after a couple of months they were divorced! I was so surprised; why leave her if she was so wonderful? The Japanese are very clever – in a sense. They never *admire* their wife or husband. So the wife always has to try to keep the husband's attention. Husbands never say, "Oh, you are beautiful!" So the wife has to work to stay attractive. Also, the wife never says, "Oh, you are wonderful!" to the husband.

It's like the brown rice taste – it's not a hot dog taste or a

Chinese restaurant taste (very spicy and oily). If you take that every day, you get tired of it. I have eaten brown rice for 40 years, and never got tired of it. If I go to a French restaurant every day, I get tired quickly. But brown rice, if cooked well, chewed well, becomes more sweet. You barely need to chew gourmet food – already it's tasty. So your marriage should be like brown rice – you have to chew very well. If you are very flashy, pretending to be like prince and princess, it doesn't last long. Better to work hard to just make a nice home; then it lasts longer.

As for choosing a partner from opposite times of birth: this type of combination has difficulties. I had a friend who married a partner with the exact opposite birthday, six months apart (she didn't know at the time, but nature did!). So Ohsawa heard about that, and was pleased. Later, the woman said, "I'm not happy; how come?" I visited her one day and found out the reason – they were opposite in hobbies and interests as well as character; they were opposite in what they wanted to do. He wanted to go out hunting, fishing; she wanted to stay at home and read. She was not interested in what he did, and he was not interested in what she did.

Ohsawa was right about opposite times of birth, but the husband and wife have to be interested in the same direction. Ohsawa married many women before Lima; Ohsawa was always interested in teaching macrobiotics to other people, but his wives were never interested in that. Only Lima-san was very much interested; she wanted to help. That's why she followed. There were many difficulties, but she was still happy following – and they had six months difference in birth.

If you have an interest in macrobiotics, you'd better have a wife who is also interested. That is more important than 'I love you' or 'You love me.' Romance may not last long, but caring lasts long. Love is a generous term, but often has certain conditions attached – 'In present conditions, I love you.' It's not absolute love, so you have to watch out. That's why many people are disappointed.

Another important thing is respect. When the husband can do something, then the wife can respect him, and when the wife can do something, the husband can respect her. Then they can last a long time. Respect means someone can do something I can't do or someone is different from me. It's different from admiration – so you don't have to be the best cook in the world. Respect is very spiritual; admiration is more sentimental, more 'flashy'. You admire the film star, but respect is *humbleness* – "She agreed to marry me, though I am not a great man." If you think, "everyone wants to marry me," then you don't respect the one who does. Humbleness in marriage is very important. Then things can be shared together. If you are haughty, then things start to break up.

Then, diet. Diet is more difficult than happiness. Most people don't know about diet in marriage. Macrobiotic people have to look after other matters, education and so on, and then diet as well – it's one more thing to think about. So it is an additional problem, or limitation, for instance in social activity. That's why I think some people quit macrobiotics; if you are very sociable, it's difficult to stay with macrobiotics – you have to compromise so often. What do you do if you are invited out by non-macrobiotic people? (George Ohsawa ate anything that was offered when he was out; then he came back home and asked us for *sho-bancha*, his medicine. He was always experimenting. But in daily diet he ate very carefully, and very little. Eating out was a good opportunity for him to try other things.)

Married couples should share interests, especially in very important matters. Modern couples, each keeping their own profession, sometimes don't last long. People used to work together, as in farming – the husband in the field, the woman looking after the home. But I had some friends who moved out to the wilderness and built a log cabin and a family from scratch. In order to make money to live, the man started a psychotherapy practice; the wife was helping too, because her father had been a famous psychologist. At first they were working together, but then she started thinking, "I can do this by myself"; then they started arguing. So finally they separated, now with separate businesses.

Why do the families of so many macrobiotic teachers break up even though they have followed all this? Maybe for other reasons. Maybe they are expecting too much, asking too much – especially the macrobiotic boy who wants a perfect macrobiotic wife, a perfect example of the human being. Men especially seem to look idealistically at women.

In Japan, maybe 90 percent of marriages were family (arranged) marriages, like Charles and Diana – not individual marriages. The kind of family you come from is very important. If there is equal income, then it is a good match. Also they check job and education – the mediator checks this first; they also check, for three generations, history of suicide, disease, etc. It's a very close examination. Then the couple meet if it is arranged, and talk about hobbies and interests. Then, if they like each other, they go ahead and marry. They respect the advice; advice is very weighty. Young people have no experience, so they rely on the recommendations of their mediator who knows both families and both sides well.

Even so, within a year – in any marriage – there is going to be fighting and crisis. In this type of arranged marriage, there is someone to go to – the mediator; he can talk to the wife or husband and maybe they can go back together. The mediator can be available for many years, because mother or father is not so good – too much personal feeling. A third person is very important; objective, like a marriage counselor. (But a professional marriage counselor doesn't know the families, so it's not as good.) Some mediators made many marriages. Ohsawa liked to be a mediator too.

But the most important thing is a person's instinct for finding a mate – this is for the final selection. My first time in marriage, my parents advised me, though I didn't like their choice. That one didn't work. Then with Cornellia, I asked my brother to check up on her – she was in Japan, I was in New York. My brother said, "Don't marry"; she was very sick. But I said, "Yes, please come over." We had corresponded for two years. So maybe it works better not seeing the person! If you see, you are deceived. If you are only writing to each other, you cannot deceive. You cannot write lies, but you can talk lies.

Aveline loved Michio because of his writing too. Writing is very important. Talking, it is very rare to come to a serious decision; often talk is about less important things. You have to talk about what you want to achieve in your lives, find out what kind of person it is and what kind of thinking they have. The person has to be generous, so as to accept your faults and your shortcomings – they should know you are not perfect. You are not Satisfaction Guaranteed or Money Returned in Five Years. It must be a Whole Life Guarantee.

So some people are not acceptable, depending on how much you can accept. If you can accept everything, then it lasts forever. If you have reservations or conditions, then it will break up sometime. That is why people divorce – they say, So far I accept, then after that I don't. So here is a problem; many people are trying to decide – is being single better, or is being married better? Being single seems less of a problem, if they can't accept. (But then if there is less difficulty there is less happiness. Less tragedy is less joy.) You have to make a commitment to accept, then you can learn more acceptance within a marriage. I was very strict in my marriage; I was taught to be like that. Later on, I learned that I should give in more. You have to have an open, listening mind. If you can't listen, then there is no way to communicate. You have to make corrections and fix things in marriage, and know each other well; then it becomes smooth. Then you can understand each other, and it goes pretty smoothly.

For instance, Cornellia has a way of saying things that I know very well, so I can handle it well. Always when I said something, she said, "No." You have to find out how to get your wife or husband to agree with you. That takes a long time. After thirty years, I finally learned. Then it works pretty good! In marriage, both people have to try to find solutions to problems, not just one person.

To me, marriage is a test of whether your judgment is high or low. If high, it will succeed; if low, it will fail. With any husband or wife you can succeed if your judgment is good enough. Each person has different abilities, but no one has every ability. Your happiness depends on your judgment. Marriage is a very interesting challenge!

One day a young lady came to see me with her husband and daughter and son. He was not interested to see me. He only came because she asked. She wanted him to come with her because she expected that I could convince him that what she wanted him to do was right. After giving regular dietary advice to them, I talked with her alone. Then I found the real problem. She was not happy with her husband because his interests were not the same as hers.

She found excitement in conversations with other men rather than her own husband – especially on Sunday when he wanted to watch the football game on TV. For her, the football game is brutal – "not for the intelligent," she thinks, but rather for lower class people's enjoyment. So she looked at her husband with less respect, and found other men more interesting. Therefore, I told her, "You should not judge your husband's intelligence by his hobby or likings." I told her my own story.

"I like all kinds of sports, especially football games. I always watch the NFL games if I have time. I like the 49ers (I don't know why though). I always watch TV when they are playing and I am excited if they win. My daughter and wife were not interested at first. However, in 1981 the 49ers won the Super Bowl game, which made my daughter a great fan of theirs. Since then she has been a steady fan of the 49ers. My daughter and I sit in front of the TV on Sunday afternoon and show joy as well as sadness if they win or lose. As the 49ers win after competitive struggles, my daughter, who is normally very quiet, jumps up and shows great excitement. Her change in attitude made my wife, who had no knowledge of football, become interested and now she joins us to watch the game. We are all happy if the 49ers win, and sad if they lose. Our Sunday afternoon is the perfect family union and enjoyment.

"If your husband likes to watch the football game, why don't you try to find interest in it? Without that effort, your husband will never try to find interest in macrobiotics. If you are not interested in the football game, then your husband will not be interested in macrobiotics. If you want him to come to macrobiotics, you could try to become a football fan. You have to yield first, then he will come to you. Don't stand alone. Do what your husband wants to do. Then your husband will do what you want to do. That is marriage. Without such generosity, marriage will not succeed."

In modern society, people are much too ego-centered. They do not give themselves to their husband or wife. This is one cause of divorce. Personal enjoyment is less important than shared enjoyment. In my opinion, the fact that people can't give up their pleasure for their mate is one of the most important causes of divorce. Why can't they give up their pleasure? Because their judgment is low.

If we have high judgment, we will not attach ourselves to any sensorial pleasure – watching TV, interesting conversations, movies, cheesecake, wine – and thus we will never be disappointed or disillusioned to find that our mate is pursuing a pleasure different from our own. As long as we have low judgment, our marriage will bring us difficulties and troubles. And those difficulties and troubles are needed for us to improve our judgment. When we improve our judgment to the highest, our marriage is a happy one.

I can see who will make a happy marriage and who won't. But I don't say. Because when Ohsawa praised someone, that person always failed. If he said, "You are useless!" then that person succeeded. Praise creates arrogance and haughtiness – then you aren't careful every day – so it's better not to praise. Then Ohsawa started only to criticize!

So if you marry a bad man, you can succeed. If you marry a good man, you can fail. If your husband is a bad man, then you have to work harder. Marriage is a gamble – you're jumping into a jungle of lions and tigers, or an ocean of sharks. But if there's no challenge, there's no adventure!

Another thing: when you are unhappy or sick or in bad shape, that is the time you can find your *real* husband – then comes your *real* friend – not when you are happy and everything is going well.

In conclusion, I think maybe you can make two mistakes in marriage. But you'd better succeed the third time!

The Goals of Macrobiotics

The first goal of macrobiotics is to make everyone rich.

In capitalistic society, to be rich is to save enough money (or to inherit from relatives) and live from its interest.

For example, if you have saved or inherited a quarter of a million dollars, you can save it in the bank and get about $35,000 interest a year, so that your monthly income will be $2,000 – which is probably enough for a couple. If you have extra income, you add to your savings and increase the interest. In this way, your principal is always saved in the bank and you live just by the interest coming from the principal. Or instead of saving in the bank, you can invest in a good business and you may get higher interest earnings; in those, the 20 percent interest rate will be the maximum. This is being rich in the capitalistic world.

However, in the biological world, the interest rate is far advanced. (God is much more generous than bankers!)

For example, one grain of rice produces about a hundred grains, if the grain is planted in good soil and taken care of well. Therefore, in the biological world, the interest rate is ninety-nine times the principal. The interest rate is 9,900 percent, not 10 or 20 percent. So everyone who grows rice can be rich like Mr. Fukuoka (author of *The One Straw Revolution*) if he does not spoil the soil by using too many chemicals.

Eating macrobiotically means you receive this generous

God's interest. Our blood, body fluids, organs, cells, and nervous system, especially the brain, start to function as God designed. Therefore, you receive 9,900 percent interest from God. Your one dollar investment in macrobiotics will receive $99 interest, if you stay macrobiotic long enough to improve your physical and mental condition.

Almost all people who made a fortune in life starting poor lived essentially macrobiotically in youth, as their parents could not afford expensive foods. Therefore, they developed healthy bodies, smart brains, and good character so that they could make a fortune during their lifetime.

The second goal of macrobiotics is to live a long, amusing, happy life, realizing one's dreams one by one.

By living macrobiotically, you are not only living a long life, but life is very amusing because you are realizing your dream always. Most people with average incomes are trying to make money and save it for retirement, by working hard. After retirement, they enjoy what they missed by working hard before – travelling or spending time on hobbies. For them, work is not enjoyable, and they don't much want to do it. They work because they want to save their retirement money.

Macrobiotics suggests that you can make a living with what you really enjoy. Not only can you save money, but also you are loved by many people even after your death, because you are happy. Establishing such a life is the second goal of macrobiotics.

The third goal of macrobiotics is to live with freedom from financial problems. Macrobiotics guarantees freedom from financial worry, as mentioned earlier, because macrobiotic eating is so simple that the lifestyle also becomes simple. You don't eat expensive foods every day.

The macrobiotic diet makes you creative and a hard worker, as good diet increases your energy, so you will become a distinguished person in your field. This also makes you free from the fear of losing your job.

Furthermore, macrobiotics teaches us how sickness is created, as well as how to cure it; therefore, we are free from the worry of being sick. However, this will take many years of experience and understanding of macrobiotic principles.

Finally, macrobiotics aims to reach supreme judgment which makes us see that all antagonism is complementary. Macrobiotic principles can solve the problem between husbands and wives, employers and employees, capitalism vs. socialism, armaments or no armaments, etc. Of these problems, the relationship between husband and wife is probably the most common and most difficult.

If either husband or wife reaches the seventh (supreme) level of judgment, the antagonism of marriage can be solved. If one member of a family reaches the seventh level of judgment, antagonism within the family can be solved. Such a family is so happy that many other families want to learn from them how to make such a happy family.

If there were one million such families in one nation, this nation would be very happy because its rate of degenerative disease, death rate, and national medical expenditure would be low even though the General National Production and living standards were high. Their standard of living would be so high that no other country would want to fight them, but would rather learn how to become such a country. As a result, world peace could be realized without any argument.

This is the final goal of macrobiotics.

August 1984

A Unique Society
The Lama Foundation

For a long time I have wanted to visit the Lama Foundation in New Mexico, as I had heard all about its beautiful location and I thought it was a Tibetan Buddhist Center in this country. Now, Cornellia and I have had a chance to visit; we discovered that it is not a center of Tibetan Buddhism after all. However, I found it to be one of the most beautiful communities that I know of.

My dream to visit there was realized unexpectedly when I received a letter from my old friend Pat Johnson, who is now working at the Foundation, inviting Cornellia and me to teach a summer camp. I answered her immediately that we would be very happy to teach macrobiotics at the Foundation.

We flew to Albuquerque from Sacramento in the early morning; around 2:00 p.m. the big smile of Pat greeted us at the airport. After lunch in Santa Fe, Lama's beat-up, dusty, four-wheel-drive Chevy van took us via the scenic highway toward Taos, which is a famous tourist attraction and resort place in winter as well as summer. About ten miles out of Taos, a road sign said "Lama 1 mile." It is a small village with only a few houses. The Foundation is located there, so it was named Lama as well.

It was already 6:00 p.m. when we arrived after driving one mile on a dirty and bumpy road. Tired after twelve hours of air and ground travel, Cornellia and I retired to our cabin built in the woods.

276

Lama has the most beautiful scenery I have ever seen. In front of the Foundation's kitchen and dome, the whole panoramic view of the Continental Divide is spread. And in front of the Divide, we could see the cliffs of the mighty Rio Grande. There is nothing to obscure the view in front, except the mist of early morning and the darkness of night. The air is clean and there are no buildings, no electric lines, and no TV antennas.

I woke up the next morning as sunshine lit up the rustic room of our cabin. At 9:00 a.m., I went to their dome for my first lecture. It is a high and huge room that can contain a hundred people easily. The room was bright as there are many windows in the roof. I could see the vast spread of the Rocky Mountains.

About twenty-five students came to our lectures from nearby Santa Fe, Albuquerque, or Taos, and a few even came from Colorado, Texas, and Idaho. Most of them were new to macrobiotics but they were very interested. I gave lectures for six days and Cornellia gave cooking classes.

Workers at this Foundation are volunteers. They get up at 5:30 a.m.; 6:00 to 7:00 is meditation time; breakfast is at 7:00., and work starts at 8:00. At 12:00 there is lunch, and from 2:00 to 6:00 it is work again. They call this community a work community, and they work very hard. Cornelia and I wondered how they are able to do this.

Altogether there are nine buildings. All of them are kept clean, and they were built by donations. I heard that a well-known author wrote a book during his stay here, and he donated his royalties to the Foundation. This helped to build many of the buildings, including the lecture dome, kitchen building, a huge dormitory, wood workshop, and many cabins. They are working now to build an extensive study center, which is almost finished.

One of the reasons they can work so hard is their diet, which contains natural foods but is much wider than 'standard' macrobiotics; it consists of grain, vegetables, eggs, and cheese. The eggs and cheese may be necessary foods in this cold climate. The cold climate may be the main factor that makes them work so hard. In this climate, they can eat animal foods and still maintain an alkaline condition, so they work hard.

The most interesting aspects of the Foundation to me were their management and leadership. As soon as I arrived I wondered who was the leader of this place. I couldn't find any particular person, so I asked Bob Johnson, who has been my macrobiotic friend for over ten years and has lived here for the past two years, who the leader is. He said there is no leader and there are no bosses. Here, every decision is made by consensus. Therefore, sometimes it takes many hours of discussion to decide on one thing. Someone said to me that because of this consensus method, every member loses his ego gradually during the stay here. Losing one's ego seems to me to be the best education that the Lama Foundation can give; in my opinion the most important shortcoming of Westerners is their too-rigid ego, which makes them unable to cooperate with others.

But does the Lama Foundation really have no leader? It was started by two couples nineteen years ago, who came from New York. They bought one hundred acres of land and started the Foundation. But they left after living there ten years, giving the property to the Foundation, which is now governed by the volunteer workers. These volunteer workers usually stay for about two years because they then find that their life will work somewhere else. But the Foundation keeps the spirit of those volunteers. This spirit is the leader of the Foundation.

Why I Came To Earth

In macrobiotics, it is often taught that our coming into this life is coming to the center of a spiral for our present materialized form; before, our spirit was at the outside end of the spiral, in the whole infinite, immaterial area beyond it. This area is sometimes called Seventh Heaven.

So why do we come from this place, where there is no problem, to earth? I was there once; one minute of it was enough for me! I say that we come here because it is boring there. My idea is that we come here for a picnic – a picnic that may last eighty years. Here it is more interesting and you can get what you want. If you want sickness you can get sick, and if you want happiness you can get happy.

If you understand this, then you are content. If not, then you complain. Everything that we have here we chose of our own free will.

Infinity is boring. There is no Hollywood, no gossip, no complaining; everybody is satisfied. But here, everything happens very fast – like married, divorced, married, divorced! I only came for a short time, but already I stayed sixty years because it's so amusing here. I am very happy that I came to this planet. I enjoy it so much, day and night. So when I talk to my dog, Shiro, I say, "Next time, please come back as a human being." He says, "Okay."

If you are not happy it's your own fault, because you know

how to change it. Thinking there is something better than what you have is an illusion. If you are not satisfied, then make your experience better.

When I was mentally sick after my first wife committed suicide, I didn't know what to do; I lost my mind. I went to see George Ohsawa and asked to stay at his school. I did nothing. I was the laziest student. I didn't clean the house, or sell newspapers, or do anything. I was just sitting, eating, sleeping and listening to what he said, for one month. But in that time I realized what is self. I returned back to myself.

So infinity is always materializing into the center, which is our small self, and then unwinding back to infinity. This repeating rhythm makes a pulsation between the big Self and little self. Many people only take the long way there – along the spiral. But you can take a shortcut, a straight line, by prayers or contemplation. Fasting is a good way – Jesus said, "prayer and fasting" – then you have an expressway to your real Self.

If you have a big problem, then you cannot eat. If you can eat, and you think you have a problem, then your problem is not big enough. If any person can eat, then I don't worry about him. Most people don't have enough problems. God gives you more, so you can find yourself; then you are a real man.

Going back and forward like this to reach the real Self is also called reincarnation. When you die without reaching Self, then you are floating around near the center -- you cannot reach the Seventh Heaven – so you come back and try again. The Japanese say we do this seven times – maybe a lucky person does it in one time. (But I'd rather stay here.)

We can be prisoners on this planet, or else we can be prince and princess of heaven while still here on earth. So if you can be a prince, why complain? We have everything God gave us. We have freedom, but we abuse it.

When you are sick, appreciate that you have so much freedom.

George Ohsawa once told us a story. When he was in prison he helped cure many criminals. After they were released from jail, they brought back many gifts to him. Then he helped the warden cure himself, too, and the warden gave him a key. "You can leave your cell any time," he said. And when the warden went away, he always left Ohsawa in charge. So he really was free – and we are free too. We just have to realize it.

Human Relationships

There are seven stages of human relationships.

The first is the mechanical one. This is manifested simply as the yin and yang relationship, or attraction and rejection. You may feel attraction to someone without reason; such a human relationship is mechanical.

The next stage is the sensorial relationship. This type of relationship creates feeling among us. For example, someone makes us feel cool and someone else makes us feel warm. Feeling that someone is beautiful or ugly is also sensorial. Such is the second level of relationship.

Third is the emotional relationship. Liking, disliking, loving, hating, being jealous, shy, outgoing, angry, proud, timid, fearful, bold, gentle, straightforward, awkward, and so on, are emotions that human relationships create. If we live alone on an island, we will not have most of them.

The fourth is scientific, or rational. In this case, we can study or observe others objectively. This relationship, contrary to the third one, is very cool, or even alienated.

The fifth one is the social or economical relationship. In this stage, the human relationship is manifest in the form of racial, ethnic, political, or class difference.

The sixth is religious. Here the relationship is like that of a leader and the followers. The leader is not necessarily religious or spiritual, but can be a kind of hero or popular person in show business, sports, or politics.

All these relationships can further be divided into two categories; that is to say, those which are complementary and those which are antagonistic. When someone is complementary to us, we like him or love him; when someone is antagonistic to us, we dislike or even hate him. Such an emotion creates the human relationship of the enemy, the foreigner, and distance from other cultural groups.

These two kinds of human relationships were studied thousands of years ago in China by what is now described as the five element theory. The complementary arrangement was called the mother-daughter relationship, and the antagonistic arrangement was known as the destructive relationship.

The mother-daughter cycle of relationships is: Water – Wood – Fire – Soil – Metal – Water. The destructive relationships are: Water against Fire, Fire against Metal, Metal against Wood, Wood against Soil, Soil against Water. These destructive relationships are not completely antagonistic, because water may destroy fire, yet will be controlled by soil, then by wood, then by metal, then by fire. In other words, Oriental medicine teaches that relationships in this world are not only antagonistic but also complementary.

Contrary to Oriental medicine, Western science teaches the enemy concept. The concept of an enemy is the product of Western biology, which says, for instance, that the eyes of carnivorous animals are located in the front of their faces in order to find the distance between the enemy and themselves. This enemy concept created Western medicine – palliative, symptomatic medicine which considers that bacteria are our enemy. This enemy concept is the cause of war among nations, races, and cultural or religious groups. As long as we have this concept, the realization of world peace will just remain a dream.

Success in Marriage

Among human relationships, the most difficult one is the

relationship between husband and wife. The reason for this is that their relationship is so close, their egos clash easily. A couple came for consultation. In reality, the husband had no interest to see me. He came because his wife asked him to come. She wanted her husband to meet me so that I could convince him that what she is asking of her husband is right – in this case to follow a macrobiotic diet.

After I talked with wife and husband, I told the wife that she had better follow her husband, because he has better judgment, even though he doesn't agree with the macrobiotic diet. He doesn't agree with the macrobiotic diet because she does not understand the macrobiotic principle. She is too rigid and egoistic. Hearing my advice, the husband was very happy, and started to be interested in the diet.

Health. If you want to succeed in marriage, you must choose a healthy mate. If she or he is sick, the marriage will have much difficulty. If the mate is sick, the other mate will have to support, provide income, cook, and take care of children and house affairs. These will make him or her burdened and, in the long run, may cause a split. If you want to learn macrobiotic medicine, choosing such a marriage will bring a wonderful opportunity. However, be careful in selecting a sickly mate because you may end up with an unsatisfying sexual life, which is often the cause of unsuccessful marriages.

Finance. In order to succeed in marriage, the couple must have decent income or adequate financial support. Marriage without such financial support will be building a sand castle, or daydreaming. Such a marriage will collapse sooner or later. I met a couple in Toronto on a recent lecture trip. She was hesitant to marry him, even though she loved him. I found the reason, which was that he has not enough income from his present job. I advised him to change the job, which was cooking in a macrobiotic restaurant in Toronto. He agreed to take my advice. As soon as they left my consulting room, they hugged each other, and decided to marry.

Communication. The most important single factor in successful marriage is good communication between husband and wife. Also in Toronto, a wife came to see me and said that she had been unhappy with her husband because she had a feeling he was hiding something from her. Her unhappiness went away when her husband confessed that he had been smoking secretly. When he wanted to smoke he had been going somewhere else, and this made his wife suspicious. There cannot be any secret between husband and wife.

There is no better marriage than the one you have. In any marriage, there are some difficulties. Therefore, thinking that by simply changing the partner you will be happier, you may end up in another difficult marriage. It is extremely important for successful marriage that partners try to improve their communication so they can understand each other's disappointments or misunderstandings. Most of the time, bad relationships start from small and insignificant misunderstandings.

Respect. Respect for each other is a more important factor in successful marriage than love. Usually love is emotional, but respect is of a much higher consciousness and does not change as easily as love. When a couple loses respect for each other, they look at each other's shortcomings. In such a case, they cannot communicate with each other anymore and the marriage may end up in disaster. In order to have respect, both members have to try to be respected. In order to be respected, they have to maintain their original commitment, made when they first met each other, which made them want to marry. In other words, everyone has good character or excellence, which justifies being respected. We have to improve such good character or skills so that we are always able to be respected, at least by our partners.

No complaint. Complaining or nagging will create marriage breakdown, without exception. Someone who wants to succeed in marriage should not complain under any circumstances. A friend of mine always complained to her husband that he was working too much and didn't care for the family. Such complaining led the husband to find a girlfriend who did not complain. Their marriage ended in divorce. There were more reasons for the divorce, but her complaints were certainly the first cause of their marriage breakdown.

If you find something wrong with your partner, you must talk it over sincerely, without complaining. The difference between complaining and sincere talking is that complaints come from trying to protect yourself. If you talk with your whole heart, for another's benefit, your words are not complaining. Such words and talk will bring good communication and solid marriage.

Appreciation. Finally, there is one more important factor in successful marriage: that is to say, keeping an attitude of appreciation as though you are just married, even if you have been married for many years. Don't forget your husband's kind help when you were sick. Show appreciation to your wife for her devoted cooking every day, cleaning the house, washing clothes, etc. As long as you have the seed of appreciation, the marriage will be happy and last a long time. When husband and wife appreciate each other, the marriage is a success.

Peace of Mind

Nothing can bring you peace
but yourself.
Nothing can bring you peace
but the triumph of principle.

Ralph Waldo Emerson
Self Reliance

"Fifteen hundred persons had been travelling by train for several days and nights. There were eighty people in each coach. All had to lie on top of their luggage, the few remnants of their personal possessions."

Thus Viktor E. Frankl started his book, *Man's Search for Meaning* (Simon & Schuster, 1970). In this book he writes about his experience in Auschwitz. From that, he concludes that whenever one is confronted with an inescapable, awful experience in an absolutely unfree situation, one can find a freedom which exists – even in Auschwitz. He found that our happiness, sickness, and life is our responsibility, not that of our parents, doctors, or government. If we do not reach this understanding, our attitude and behavior are not happy. By realizing that he had responsibility for his happiness and well-being, he could maintain his peace of mind there.

For example, many cancer patients who ask my advice about their diet want to know how long they should stay on the strict cancer diet. They want to quit the diet as soon as the cancer becomes better. This is the result of thinking that their cancer is caused by something other than themselves. They are not being responsible for the cancer. They are observing the diet because I advised it, or merely to cure the sickness. With this attitude, they are not happy doing the diet. Since they are not happy with the diet, the diet does not give them full benefit – although as long as they follow it they will have some definite improvement. Such a person stops the diet when the cancer becomes better; then, soon they will develop another cancer. Someone who develops cancer again after curing it once will usually have much more difficulty in improving the condition the second time, even with the macrobiotic diet. These people usually give up the diet, go to medication, and terminate their life.

On the contrary, if they think that their health, happiness, and sickness are their own responsibility, they can maintain peace of mind. Since they maintain peace of mind, their organs function well and they assimilate nutrients well. The diet gives them utmost benefit. This is the stress theory of Hans Selye, and writer Norman Cousins applied the same idea in curing his own sickness. Dr. Selye detailed the negative effects of negative emotions on body chemistry.

The inevitable question arose in my mind: what about the positive emotions? If negative emotions produce negative chemical changes in the body, wouldn't positive emotions produce positive chemical changes? Thus, Cousins applied laughter therapy and Selye recommends gratitude as an important stress-solving mentality. George Ohsawa told us that absolute faith in the order of the universe will bring us to Seventh Heaven. Peace of mind does the same thing. This peace of mind will be ours if we take responsibility for our deeds as well as our health, sickness, success, or failure.

Next to responsibility, the condition which brings us a

peaceful mind is 'no jealousy'. Jealousy is the incapability of admitting the success of others or our own failure. This is negative emotion. This destroys peace of mind and makes us nervous, irritable, unstable, and unhappy. There is jealousy in all of the competitive world, such as business, sports, show businesss, and even the scholarly world. Any competition may cause jealousy. Therefore, in order to avoid jealousy, it is best not to be competitive. However, competitiveness is positive emotion, while jealousy is negative emotion. Competitiveness itself can help us to develop and grow. It is not a bad emotion. However, it can turn to jealousy, which is destructive of peace of mind – a more important thing to acquire than money, prestige, fame, or success in any field. Many people exchange peace of mind for those vanities. This is the pit into which many distinguished people, even the greatest spiritual leaders, may fall.

About a thousand years ago, Japan produced two of her most distinguished Buddhist monks. They were Saicho of the Tendai sect and Kukai of the Shingon sect. Both of them were selected as exchange students by the Japanese Emperor at that time, and went to China by small boats when they were very young. Saicho founded the Japanese Tendai sect on Mt. Hiei, near Kyoto. He was their greatest teacher. He had many distinguished disciples who started three of the most popular Buddhist schools, namely the Shin sect by Shinran, the Soto Zen sect by Dogen, and the Nichiren sect by Nichiren. He was considered the best teacher of Japanese Buddhism at that time. Even the Emperor studied with him.

On the other hand, Kukai learned Tibeten Esoteric Buddhism after living inland in the far west of China. He established the Shingon sect at the top of Mt. Koyo. He never cultivated great disciples; however, he made himself a most popular Buddhist monk by teaching farmers, villagers, merchants and other lower class people how to build bridges, how to control floods, how to make rice fields, and other practical matters.

These two Buddhist monks who distinguished themselves by their character, philosophy, and way of teaching became some of the most fierce rivals and competitors in Japanese Buddhism. They argued on the theory of Buddhism publicly and officially. One day, Saicho wrote a letter to Kukai in which he asked to borrow a book on esoteric Buddhism which Kukai had brought back from China. In a letter of reply, Kukai said no. Even such a great man and spiritual leader couldn't resist antagonistic competitiveness. Although I don't know whether Kukai refused to lend the book to Saicho from jealousy or not, this story shows us how difficult it is to reach a mentality in which we have no competitiveness or jealousy. For this reason, Ohsawa taught us that we should graduate from the business world at the age of forty or so.

In fact, I quit business much younger when I was in New York because I didn't like the competitiveness of the business world. Around 1956, I started a retail store in midtown Manhattan. Soon Michio and other macrobiotic friends started similar stores. Friends until then, we became business enemies, or competitors. I didn't like the emotion created by that competitiveness. So I sold my share of the store to my partner, and I moved to California. Since then, I never became involved with competitive business. This new attitude brought me peace of mind.

Pursuing fame and status creates jealousy, and then loss of peace of mind. Therefore, Lao Tsu warned us not to be too much concerned with fame or the desire to reach high status:

> People are too concerned with fame and shame.
> People are giving too much value to their ego desires
>   instead of the desires that come from the inner self.
> What do I mean by saying people are too concerned
>   with fame?

It means that people want fame and not shame, by any means.

They are so depressed when they gain shame or lose fame.

What do I mean by saying that people give too much value to their ego desires?

When people give too much value to their ego desires, they acquire sickness.

Therefore elimination of ego desire is the cure of sickness.

One who is concerned with the real self but not ephemeral ego desire can be trusted.

One who loves the eternal self and not the temporal self – such as fame and prestige – can be relied on.

Tao Tou
Tao Teh Ching
(Chapter 13)

Ohsawa's
Macrobiotic Spirit

In order to understand macrobiotics, we must understand Ohsawa's spirit. His spirit and thinking was influenced chiefly by five aspects: Bushi-Dō or Samurai-Dō, Buddhism, Yin Yang philosophy, the teachings of Ishizuka, and his mother's example.

Bushi-Dō

Ohsawa's concept of life or lifestyle came from the samurai spirit. He taught living with an all-or-nothing attitude; he believed and taught that the foundation of health and happiness is always to endure such things as cold and hunger. He believed that cold and hunger (both yin) will produce physiological and spiritual yang and that health is the only weapon we can rely on to reach happiness in this ever-changing world.

His second concept of life also comes from Bushi-Dō, that is to say, he did not allow making any excuse. He learned the no-excuse attitude of the samurai from his mother – not from his father who was a samurai. One day his mother pushed him to the ground by accident and he was injured. She never made any excuse for her mistake; she apologized to her husband by complete surrender. She waited for her husband to return home, and expected him to punish her with his samurai sword.

Ohsawa believed that excuses are the foundation of Western civilization – demonstrated by lawyers, contracts, politics, and medicine. All offer excuses for violating natural law.

Ohsawa taught that someone who makes excuses for their mistakes never learns from them, and therefore will never become a happy man. He scolded his students if they made excuses for their mistakes. Such education often made his students leave him. However, many appreciated such education later, because they learned that an excuse is ego protestation, and as long as we live with ego protestation we are not happy. However, Ohsawa did not give the education of 'no excuse' as much to the Western people as he did to the Japanese. Ohsawa knew it was too much to ask at the beginning.

The next important concept that comes from Bushi-Dō is the idea of justice. He considered that to live with justice or absolute honesty is the highest stage of health. Then what is justice? According to Ohsawa, justice is 'everything changes' – the order of the universe. That is to say, this world is made of yin and yang; yin changes to yang, yang changes to yin and so on. The macrobiotic diet and medicine, therefore, are based on the order of the universe. Furthermore, his diet and medicine, and the whole of macrobiotics, is nothing but a way of education toward understanding absolute justice, all-embracing love, and eternal faith. He didn't care about symptomatic cures, because they do not teach justice or real happiness. What he really wanted to teach was how people can develop real, not superficial, happiness.

When he was in France, a young man came to see him one day. It was his son, who had grown up without him as father. This son had been bitten by a poisonous snake and he became very sick. Instead of consoling him, Ohsawa scolded him very severely. He wanted his son to understand justice: that sickness is the punishment of God, given to those who disobey justice. For the same reason, Ohsawa refused to help cure anybody he had once helped. He thought that real curing is following or understanding justice. If someone becomes sick

again, it means that he did not understand the original cause of
the sickness. Therefore, it was no use to help the person again,
because it would not bring understanding of justice or real
health. This was his education and the education of macrobiotics.

Zen Buddhism

Ohsawa spent some of his childhood years in a Zen temple.
He must have recalled the Zen monks' diet when he first
learned about Ishizuka's diet. Without the experience of the
temple, he might not have been interested in Ishizuka's diet at
all. The Buddhist diet originally emphasized avoiding animal
foods. Ohsawa repeatedly said that man can live without any
animal foods. Recent nutritional study is confirming this, but
his thought came not from nutritional theory but from
Buddhism.

The philosophy of macrobiotics is greatly influenced by
Buddhism. For example, Ohsawa's first book in French, *The
Unique Principle,* contains Shinran's *Tannisho* translation.
Ohsawa often quoted words from the *Tannisho:* "Everything
in this world is vanity, ephemeral, and relative; there is no
truth." This concept led him to search for truth naturally. In
the same book, Ohsawa translated the *Hannya Hara Mitta
Shin Gyo,* which describes the character of infinity, reality, and
the absolute, or the world of no change – the world of truth and
justice. These two concepts, the world of the relative and the
world of truth, led him to the revolutionary concept of the
order of the universe, in which he unified the relative world
with the world of the absolute, or God. His creation of the
concept of the order of the universe is the greatest work in
man's history. With this concept, anyone who is seriously
seeking God or peace can be guided there. Ohsawa wrote this
concept for the first time in *The Order of the Universe* (not yet
published in English), which he thought was the most important book he ever wrote.

Yin Yang Philosophy

The concept of yin and yang is not Ohsawa's creation; it is an age-old idea from the East. Therefore, it is not coincident that he was interested in this concept when he was young. He said in *The Unique Principle* that he learned about the *I-Ching* from a friend. Study of the *I-Ching* made him realize that everything in this world changes through yin-and-yang order. He never stopped thinking. He united the yin-and-yang changing world with the *Hannya Shin Gyo*'s no-change world. According to him, there are six yin-and-yang worlds and they are all parts of one world, infinity. Later he improved this idea by introducing the spiralic concept. He created a graphic explanation of the world, starting with infinity and going through yin and yang polarity; energy; pre-atomic matter; minerals; the plant world; and the animal world.

Sagen Ishizuka's Diet

Ohsawa was diagnosed with tuberculosis when he was eighteen years old. Given up by doctors, he searched outside orthodox medicine. At that time, he came across a book written by Dr. Sagen Ishizuka, teaching about a grain and vegetable diet and the potassium/sodium balance. Observing Ishizuka's diet, Ohsawa cured his tuberculosis in two years. Since then, Ohsawa devoted himself to spreading the teachings of Ishizuka, which consisted of five principles: 1. Foods are the origin or source of life; without food there is no life. 2. The main food for mankind is grain. 3. One should eat locally grown and seasonal foods. 4. Whole and unrefined foods are foods for health. 5. The potassium and sodium ratio must be kept to a certain proportion.

After many years of studying and teaching Ishizuka's diet, Ohsawa changed "potassium-and-sodium proportion" to "yin-and-yang proportion," and named the diet "macrobiotic."

Ohsawa not only established the macrobiotic diet but also macrobiotic principles and philosophy.

Mother's Influence

One day at a seminar in Tokyo, around 1963, Ohsawa talked about his mother as his lifelong educator.

"My mother was divorced from my father when she was twenty-five, after five years of marriage. Then she studied nursing and midwifery at the Dō-Shi-Sha University in order to support her family. After graduating, she was busy helping the sick and poor. Thus, her attitude made me work hard for the sick and poor later. However, within her character the most important thing was that she never complained of her sickness, her husband's lack of integrity or financial difficulties, or anything else.

"After five years of hard work, she contracted tuberculosis, probably due to her bad diet learned from Western nutritional theory. When the sickness was very advanced, she called her two surviving sons to her bedside. She told me to become a scholar because I was yin, and directed my young brother to become a soldier because he was yang. After telling us about our future, she lay in bed quietly for about thirty minutes, and died. She never cried or complained, even though she worried about the future of her two sons, resenting my father's unfaithful conduct. She was concerned about the family's poor financial situation.

"This is education. People often talk too much. Then they cannot impress lifelong virtues or attitudes on others. My mother taught me 'don't complain' without words, when she was dying. Therefore, I followed it for sixty years, and by this teaching I could change thousands of people to macrobiotics. What I am now, and want to be in the future, is influenced by my mother who died when I was ten."

Holding On and Letting Go
Address at French Meadows Summer Camp

I would like to tell you about when I was first studying from George Ohsawa.

Ohsawa taught me orderliness. He came to New York in 1959 and began lecturing in 1960. He gave lectures about distinguished people and when their birthdays occurred – Van Gogh, Anatole France, Gandhi, Jesus Christ. Revolutionaries are born in May, also artists in May, but musicians in winter. (Van Gogh was crazy – too yang!)

I wrote down his lectures as he talked, and published them in our newsletter. Then he scolded me very much, because I didn't put any order in them – I published them just as he lectured, month by month. He didn't accept any excuse from me.

That was the biggest education he offered – no excuse. Nature doesn't accept excuses. But our mother and father do, so we grow up learning how to make them. So Ohsawa tried to show the mistake of accepting the concept of excuses and taking it for granted. If we do that, then our accumulation of mistakes becomes very great.

Ohsawa scolded his students very much. But I am sentimental – I cannot scold. I am too weak to scold, even if I see unhappiness coming for someone. I let them find out for themselves. Then God does justice. I don't need to do anything. Everyone wants to be popular. No one wants to be a bad guy. I am like that – I always wanted to be liked. I never said bad things about others, or hated them. So nobody disliked me. (But I don't like lazy people, because when they are around I can't get any rest.) But I admire people who let themselves be hated. They are very wonderful, very great men. Like Jesus Christ, such guys are the most important people.

If you like someone, then they are the opposite of you. If you hate someone, it is because they are like you. Understanding this makes relationships very smooth.

One time I lived in Sacramento. We always had visitors, including hippies. Cornellia didn't like them – they made her very busy, especially the lazy ones. One time she complained about one guy. I said, "We better keep him because then no other lazy guys will come. One lazy guy is enough in the home, then another one doesn't want to come." She understood, and happily kept him.

Likewise, if you're sick, don't cure yourself – it's no good to be perfect. And the same way, everyone wants a perfect marriage. That's why there are so many divorces in this country.

How to think in these opposites is macrobiotics. There are always two kinds of view. If one view doesn't make you happy, then change to another.

I used to like fishing very much, with my family. Then the family lost interest, so I gave up fishing and my enjoyment of it. Sometimes you have to give in; especially for the family, you have to learn to give up. But actually, in life, happiness comes when you give things up. Happiness doesn't come when you hold on.

For instance, when you start macrobiotics, you are very happy because you gave up meat or cheese. Then, when you like brown rice and miso soup, you have to give them up. Many people are unhappy because they're stuck to brown rice and miso. When you cure sickness using brown rice, it's not only the brown rice that cures you but also what you gave up. So the next time you get sick, it's almost incurable because then you only have brown rice, miso, and soy sauce to give up!

If you master this relationship, you can be very happy. I smoked for twenty-five years, so I gave it up – because I liked it. So if you like your husband, give him up; then he stays with you. Otherwise, you will lose him. And if you hold on to health, you lose it.

All great teachers were at one time very miserable. What they learned was detaching from ego, and getting to the big Self. If you give up ego, you lose nothing. But it is very difficult. Most unhappy people I meet are unhappy because of this attachment. Yet giving it up is the easiest thing to do, too. Still, you can only do what you want to do, but be ready to give it up.

Most people make rules – I should do this, or I should do that. Become like water; it fits whatever container you put it in. If your mind is one shape, then it is too rigid. What we like is the opposite of what we are. This is how relationships work.

When I left my family, I didn't tell them I was going. But my mother knew. She made me a meal. It was mochi with sugar, so I didn't eat it. That was the last meal she made for me. I never saw her again. I still regret not eating it. Since then, I have eaten cakes with sugar many times – so why not eat hers? Stupidity. Rigidity. As if I loved macrobiotics more than her, or loved myself more than her.

So please be careful to always develop the bigger Self. The macrobiotic tendency is the opposite. Don't exchange brown rice for happiness.

December 1984

Real Health

The ultimate goal of macrobiotics is to attain real health, eternal happiness, and non-exclusive justice. George Ohsawa demonstrated this when he visited Albert Schweitzer. He deliberately acquired the tropical ulcer disease in order to show how the macrobiotic diet can cure a sickness Schweitzer believed incurable. To Ohsawa, observing the macrobiotic diet is following the order of the universe, and so it is justice.

Ohsawa compiled six conditions of health at the age of thirty-nine. Thirty years later he added a seventh condition, far more important than the other six. [*Ed.:* See "The Seventh Condition of Health," page 74.] The seven conditions of health as I teach them are:

Physical conditions
1. Never being tired.
2. Good, deep sleep.
3. Good appetite.

Psychological conditions
4. Freedom from anger.
5. No complaining.

Spiritual conditions
6. Deep appreciation for everything, even failures.
7. Absolute faith in justice – the order of the universe.

Since behavior is preceded by attitude, the above conditions of health are preceded by attitudes. The three physiological conditions are the result of an attitude of trying to observe the macrobiotic diet, which produces behavior corresponding to the macrobiotic diet. Then, the attitude which will bring us the fourth condition of health, no anger, is the commitment, "I will not be angry under any circumstances." The attitude which brings us the fifth condition of health, not complaining, is taking responsibility. Someone who takes responsibility under any circumstances will not complain, even when his wishes or desires are not realized. He keeps his peace of mind even when he is surrounded by disappointment, failure, and antagonism.

The difference between macrobiotic medicine and modern medicine is in whether one takes responsibility or not. In the view of macrobiotic medicine, one has responsibility for his sickness; in modern medicine, bacteria or viruses are given responsibility for causing it. Therefore, one who doesn't think he is responsible for his sickness will not cure it even though he observes the diet seriously. In other words, if one's mentality is not right, the body's metabolism, chemical reactions, and organ functions will not perform according to their highest order.

What makes one appreciative is to always keep one's hunger. If we are hungry, we appreciate meals. If this behavior is repeated, we become appreciative all the time. But the cultivation of the behavior of living with justice is not easy. And this is best done before one reaches six years of age; in other words, one learns this attitude from a mother who never tells lies.

In order to understand the concept of true health, one must understand that real health does not exist in the relative world. There are several concepts which cannot be seen, heard, or told; justice or health are such concepts. Freedom, happiness, life, peace, eternity, harmony, integrity, beauty, and truth are all concepts which nobody has adequately explained. Everybody wants them, but instead they find and stay with their opposites – unhappiness, death, sickness, quarrels, war, ugliness, lies, anger, hate – which only make them unhappy, unfree, and unjust in the end.

The health which most people wish to have is only relative to sickness. In other words, such health is always turning into sickness, and vice versa. Therefore, having such health is not our ultimate aim. The ultimate aim of health is eternal health. Then, what is eternal health? Can we get it?

Yes, we can. Eternal health includes relative health and sickness. Since it includes sickness, it includes eternity, totality, and truth. George Ohsawa contracted tropical ulcers and cured it. This is real health.

When you are healthy you are attracted to goodies such as ice cream, peaches, beer, and so on. You eat these eventually – a little at first, then a little more. If your health is not immediately affected by them, then you increase the consumption. One day you have headaches or stomachaches. This is relative health and relative sickness. Attaining such health does not bring you peace of mind. You are always afraid to be sick. You follow macrobiotics because of fear. Then you are a fearful person. You are not healthy at all. Such is not the goal of macrobiotics.

The goal of macrobiotics is to attain eternal health. Eternal health includes relative health and relative sickness. Knowing you can be sick sometimes and knowing how to cure it is real health. When you are sick, you know how you caused the sickness, and you reflect upon your own mistakes and commit that you will not make the same mistake again.

In other words, real health is the judgment or understanding of the law of the changing world. For someone who has this judgment or understanding, his consciousness is outside of relativity. It is in the eternal world. This is real health or eternal health, and the ultimate goal of macrobiotics.

Since the eternal world is only one, eternal health is another name for real happiness, truth, love, or peace. When we reach this understanding, we understand the meaning of our life. We understand why we come to this planet called Earth. We are so joyful that we cry.

January 1985

Happy New Year 1985

The macrobiotic movement in the United States began in New York City when George Ohsawa gave the first seminars on macrobiotics in January of 1960. Since then, a quarter of a century has passed. On the occasion of the New Year celebration, it may be worthwhile to recall the spirit of Ohsawa – that is to say, what his motivation was in starting to teach macrobiotics.

When Ohsawa was six years old, his father left his home for a girlfriend. Caring for George and his younger brother and sister, their mother didn't know how to live. She lost her mind. However, this strong-minded mother was able to recover from depression. She studied nursing and midwifery and got a license.

She worked hard in helping sick and pregnant women. She gave free help if patients were poor. However, the hard work caused her to become sick; she became infected with tuberculosis germs from a patient. She was afraid that the disease might be passed on to her children, and her sickness cut off the family income. Their home became so poor that they could hardly eat. Knowing she was going to die soon, she worried about her children's future. But she never complained, and never allowed her children to complain either. She died after six months of fighting the disease on June 17, 1903 at the age of thirty-two. George Ohsawa was then ten years old. His mother's death was a tremendous shock and had an impact on his whole life. Ohsawa vowed to his mother that he would fight the diseases that can kill a young mother, leaving helpless children behind. He knew what it was to suffer because of a mother's sickness. Therefore, Ohsawa wanted to work through his whole life to bring the day when no young mother would suffer from any disease. This is the spirit in which Ohsawa founded macrobiotics.

However, for his spirit to form the macrobiotic diet, he needed another experience. He himself acquired tuberculosis, and the sickness led him to find Sagen Ishizuka and his diet (the natural diet, *shoku-yo* in Japanese). As soon as he cured his tuberculosis with the diet, he decided to spread knowledge of it so that young mothers like his own would not die anymore and have to worry about the future of their sons and daughters.

Ohsawa followed the wordless teaching of his mother – no complaining, study all the time, cure the sick. However, there was one difference between his and his mother's work. Ohsawa cured the sick by the macrobiotic diet, and his mother tried to cure with Western nursing and nutrition. Ohsawa helped the sick, giving lectures, consultations, and even treatments for over twenty years. He cured thousands of sick people. He realized the tremendous curing power of the macrobiotic diet, which most doctors, nurses, and even the sick – who were cured by the diet – did not realize.

He also realized the uselessness of curing the sick, because there are always sick people no matter how many are cured. After World War II, he stopped curing the sick; instead, he started to teach macrobiotic philosophy and diet and way of life. In other words, he changed the direction of the macrobiotic movement from curing sickness to education about diet and philosophy.

In the United States, therefore, he started teaching this, and curing the sick was not emphasized. When Dr. Sattilaro cured his cancer, the macrobiotic diet was recognized as medicine. Now most people are starting the diet because of their wish to cure sickness. This is the situation of macrobiotics in the United States today. In other words, the macrobiotic movement in the United States is in the situation of the 1920s, 1930s, and 1940s in Japan. Most Americans are not interested in macrobiotics, but there are sick persons who are only interested because it may cure their sickness.

Since politics in the United States at present is very similar to that of the military politics around the beginning of this century in Japan, the United States may get involved in a third world war. Even if we can avoid the catastrophe of war, foods supplied in this country may eventually sentence most of the population to cancer and wipe out the people who follow the advertisements of TV, magazines, and regular school education. This will happen within twenty years, unless the world leaders of today realize the importance of health and peace of mind. Macrobiotic students who survive such destruction will be the leaders of the new age which is coming.

In any case, we should stop such destruction by any means possible. Like George Ohsawa who couldn't stop Japan's involvement in the war, we may not be able to stop the coming catastrophe of war and the cancer epidemic; but let us students of macrobiotics recall the spirit of Ohsawa and work harder to educate the public about macrobiotic philosophy and diet – the principle of peace – this year, which is a quarter of a century after the first teaching of macrobiotics began in this country.

The Disastrous
Macrobiotic Diet

In the October 17, 1984 edition of the *Bellingham Herald* the following question was asked: "A friend says she has read that macrobiotic diets can successfully treat cancer. Is there any evidence to support her claim?"

In response, Dr. Jean Mayer, president of Tufts University and the holder of several doctorate degrees in nutrition, replied plainly:

> No. While macrobiotic literature contains reports of miraculous cures by diet, there have been no reports in medical journals describing the course of cancer patients following these diets, nor have there been any controlled studies of the diet in suitable animal cancer models.
>
> The macrobiotic theory of disease sees 'a cancer as an attempt on the part of the organism to create a balance. If the cancer is removed, this overall balance will be disrupted and collapse.' To maintain harmony, this 'natural' phenomenon should not be disrupted either by removing or destroying it. Thus, macrobiotics advocates diet as the main therapy for cancer.
>
> This is downright disastrous. Proper nutritional management is an essential adjunct in treating cancer patients, but is never the main therapy.

I agree with Dr. Mayer: the macrobiotic cancer diet is disastrous. It is disastrous in the sense that any diet or treatment, including the macrobiotic approach, is as disastrous as conventional cancer treatment, because we do not know what the cause of cancer is, or the exact mechanism that causes normal cells to change to malignant cells and malignant cells to develop. Until we know exactly the cause and mechanism of cancer development, any treatment or therapy is disastrous – including surgery, radiation, and chemotherapy.

In my opinion, cancer cells are irreversible. In other words, cancer cells can't change back to normal cells again. Once normal cells have become malignant, they do not change, even with the macrobiotic diet.

For this reason, while the official therapy for cancer is to remove it or attempt to kill the cancer cells, the aim of the macrobiotic approach is to stop further growth of the cancer cells until they eventually die out. In order to do this, macrobiotics tries to discourage any further cancer cell development by restricting or limiting the caloric protein intake. Due to this, Dr. Mayer thinks the macrobiotic diet is a hindrance to curing cancer. ("Because patients with weight loss have a poorer prognosis, concern about the caloric adequacy of these diets is clearly justified . . . . Especially for those who are losing weight, protein intake may be insufficient.") But here is the doctor's misunderstanding. The macrobiotic diet is not for curing cancer. In fact, no diet can cure cancer and no treatment can cure cancer. We can only stop its development. In order to do so, we have to limit the supply of protein, as it encourages further development of cancer cells.

Since there is no absolute cure for cancer, danger or even disaster exists in any therapy or diet. It is just a matter of choice as to which way to go – the macrobiotic way, or surgery, radiation, or chemotherapy. The macrobiotic way is to stop the further development of cancer, which may cause weight loss, whereas conventional medicine tries to destroy cancer cells, with the danger of also destroying many normal cells.

There are some advantages in conventional treatment (even though it destroys normal cells) if one's digestive and circulatory functions are not good, which means that the dietary approach may not work well. The article by Dr. Mayer points out that the complex carbohydrates and fiber in cereal grains may be less easily digested and absorbed by certain cancer patients. But if one has good digestive and circulatory systems, the macrobiotic diet works very well. However, we do not consider even this to be therapy because we are not curing cancer cells. The macrobiotic approach is prevention of cancer cell development and even malignant cell formation.

Considering these differences between macrobiotics and conventional medicine, Dr. Mayer is right in a sense but has missed the point of what the macrobiotic diet is trying to do. In conclusion, I say again that the macrobiotic diet is preventive of cancer, and not therapy. The macrobiotic diet, in my opinion, prevents cancer well, even after malignant cells have been produced. But it is not therapy. Therefore, it is not to be compared with treatments such as surgery, radiation, or chemotherapy.

April 1985

What is Yin and Yang?

One night during a recent Vega class a lady asked me, "If I am yin now, how can I be yang later?" I answered, "Because everything changes. Yin has to change to yang because there are only yin and yang in this world." However, she was still in doubt. I wondered why she could not comprehend this reasoning. I felt that there must be something wrong with our teaching that caused confusion in the explanation of yin and yang. Or there was some difference between her understanding of yin and yang and my understanding of the concept. After thinking about this matter for awhile, I finally understood the difference. It was that she thought of yin and yang as names given to things, and I think of them as adjectives. For her if she is called yin, then her name is Yin, and therefore she is Yin for her whole life. I explained that the words 'yin' and 'yang' are merely adjectives which modify nouns, nouns which can name anything – humans, animals, and anything we can think, see, hear, smell, taste, and touch.

For instance, we say this is a beautiful flower. The word 'beautiful' is an adjective which describes the condition of the flower at that time. The same flower may not be beautiful tomorrow. Then we will call the flower ugly. Yin and yang are also adjectives which describe the conditions of various things, including abstract things. The flower does not change its nature, so its name does not change. But the condition of the flower changes, and so do the adjectives, the describing words.

The student seemed to understand yin and yang better. But then I was reading in Ohsawa's books and I found that he was using the words 'yin' and 'yang' as nouns. And not only that, he explained yin and yang with several meanings, none of them clear for most beginners of macrobiotics. For example, in *The Book of Judgment* (G.O.M.F., 1980), he uses them as classifiers:

> The unique principle divides all things into two antagonistic categories: Yin and Yang, according to the Chinese wise men, or Tamasic and Rajasic, if one follows the Indian saints. . . . They are indeed two complementary forces indispensable to each other, like man to woman or day to night. They are the two fundamental and opposite factors that continually produce, destroy and produce, repeatedly, all that exists in the universe. Yin and yang exist in everything on an infinitely diversified scale.

In his book *Zen Macrobiotics* (Ohsawa Foundation, 1965) the explanation is the same.

The philosophical concept or idea of yin and yang began in China. It was first stated in the *I-Ching*. According to the *I-Ching*, yin and yang are two poles of infinity, and the combinations of these two poles make four states of yin and yang. By adding one more yin and yang factor to the four states it is possible to come up with eight combinations. And finally, by combining those eight trigrams, the *I-Ching* makes sixty-four hexagrams. With these symbols the *I-Ching* has been used as a book of divination for thousands of years.

In the *I-Ching* it is not clear what yin and yang are except that they are two sides of infinity. George Ohsawa probably learned the spiralic form of the creation of the universe from the *I-Ching*. He said that infinity manifests itself when yin and yang divide and produce in turn: energy, then particles, elements, the world of plants, and finally the animal world. This spiralic pattern can be pictured as follows:

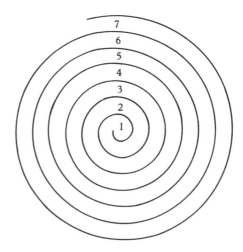

7. Infinity
6. Yin Yang Polarity
5. Vibration-Energy
4. Pre-Atomic Particles
3. Elements
2. Plants
1. Animals

Five of these seven regions of the spiral can themselves be divided into seven 'worlds' as follows:

The Vibration-energy level
      7th Magnetism (transition to/from yin yang polarity)
▽ 6th Light
△ 5th Electricity
▽ 4th Heat
△ 3rd Chemical Energy
▽ 2nd Mechanical Energy
△ 1st Gravity

The Pre-atomic world
      7th Photon (transition to/from the vibration-energy level)
▽ 6th Electron
△ 5th Neutrino
▽ 4th Lambda
△ 3rd Neutron
▽ 2nd Sigma
△ 1st Proton

The world of Elements

    7th H (transition to/from the pre-atomic world)

▽ 6th He, Ne, Ar, Kr, Xe, Rn

△ 5th Li, Be, Na, Mg, K, Ca

▽ 4th Ti, V, Cr, Mn, F, Co, Ni, Cu, Zn, Mo, W, Pt, Au, Hg

△ 3rd B, C, Al, Si

▽ 2nd N, O, P, S, As

△ 1st Fe, Cl, Br, I, At

The world of Plants

    7th Seed (transition to/from the world of elements)

▽ 6th Fruit

△ 5th Flower

▽ 4th Leaf

△ 3rd Branch

▽ 2nd Stem

△ 1st Root

The Animal world

    7th Plankton (transition to/from the world of plants)

▽ 6th Shellfish

△ 5th Fish

▽ 4th Reptile

△ 3rd Bird

▽ 2nd Mammal

△ 1st Human being

This is the constitution of the world as George Ohsawa taught it to us. As you have probably realized by now, yin and yang are two constitutional forces existing in everything, from the world of energy to the world of animal life. Yin and yang also exist in nonliving things, in abstract concepts, emotions, and spiritual activities. Yin and yang, then, may be used to classify all phenomena according to the degree of their manifestation of yin-yang strength at any particular moment. At the beginning of macrobiotic study, however, the richness of this classification system is not only difficult but also confusing. Because of this I recommend that beginners think of the words 'yin' and 'yang' as adjectives – words which describe the changing conditions of things, people, thoughts, and other phenomena.

Ohsawa Is Coming

"Ohsawa is coming! Ohsawa is coming!" Those were the words most often repeated among the macrobiotic folk in New York City in November of 1959. There were about six of Ohsawa's students living there at the time, and six or seven more living in other parts of the United States.

We talked about Ohsawa's coming and were afraid that we were in for one of his severe scoldings because we hadn't been doing any macrobiotic work. Instead we had been operating our own retail shops on the busy streets of New York.

Ohsawa arrived at Pier 34 during the last days of 1959. Since I was the only one who was free to pick him up, he chose my home to stay in. He was about sixty-six years old then and we were all happy that he was not as severe as he had been as a younger man.

He was at my place just long enough to stretch his legs when he flew to the West Coast. He came back a couple of weeks later with information about California brown rice and stories of his meeting in Los Angeles with his old friend Paul Richard. This was the first we had known of brown rice in America; Ohsawa had to come from France in order to find it for us.

In January, 1960 he began a series of lectures in a room I had rented in the Buddhist Academy, then headed by Reverend Seki, on Riverside Drive. Ohsawa was asked to repeat the lecture series and during the second and third series Lima

315

Ohsawa held cooking classes in the kitchen. She held classes, the students ate, and then Ohsawa lectured.

Ohsawa's main aim was to improve the quickness and soundness of his students' thinking. For example, after he had explained about yin and yang, he took questions about anything – nutrition, biology, physiology, psychology, social problems, religion, the news of the day, even politics. He always welcomed the students' questions. His lectures were full of wit and humor and his audience laughed a great deal. The class was full of the joy of learning, even with such difficult subjects as how to be happy in any circumstances.

Each of Ohsawa's lectures began with daily topics. He would ask the students for their thoughts and opinions on these topics and after they had spoken he would give his own thoughts and criticisms on what they had said. He always started his lectures with materialistic subjects and ended with spiritual subjects, another way in which Ohsawa demonstrated excellent teaching ability.

Ohsawa's greatest concern was that we understand and live with Oneness or Infinity. In other words, he wanted us to live without exclusivity. He wanted us to accept everything with joy and appreciation, making no excuses for ourselves. Most of the students improved their thinking ability and gained a much better understanding of Ohsawa's teachings on the order of the universe and happiness.

Since those first American lectures, twenty-five years have gone by, and during that time macrobiotics in this country almost died once due to bad publicity. However, after having experienced many difficulties, it has survived. And the reason is simple. The macrobiotic teaching is needed in this suffering and confused America, and in the whole world as well. As long as people are suffering from incurable sicknesses and are living in a helpless state of emotional turmoil, the macrobiotic teaching will continue to offer an alternative.

June 1985

Sexually Transmitted Disease

The United States, one of the most affluent societies in the world, is experiencing an epidemic rise in glamorous and fashionable diseases which are all related to sexual contact – that is to say, sexually transmitted diseases, or STD. Recently I have been studying these diseases from the point of view of macrobiotics, and I have discovered some very interesting things.

According to the Center for Disease Control in Atlanta, Georgia, as reported in the February 4, 1985 issue of *Newsweek*, the estimated numbers of new cases of STD in 1984 alone were as follows:

Chlamydia	3,000,000
Gonorrhea	2,000,000
Venereal Warts	1,000,000
Herpes	500,000
Syphilis	90,000
AIDS	4,500

As the figures show, the fastest spreading STD of today is chlamydia, which struck about three million Americans of both sexes last year alone. (One reason chlamydia was diagnosed so much last year is that scientists have recently found an easy way to diagnose the disease. Until then, it had been very difficult to diagnose.) The first symptoms of chlamydia are deceptively gentle: simple infection, a slight discharge, and mild pain.

It seems to me that the microorganisms of chlamydia are yang, and some can survive the protective attack of our antimicrobial immune system. The surviving chlamydia frequently move to the uterine lining and the Fallopian tubes, causing pelvic inflammation disease or PID. This can cause blockage of the Fallopian tubes, which is one of the most serious forms of STD.

Increasing its number of victims by two million in 1984, gonorrhea was the second most active STD in this country. Syphilis, with only 90,000 new victims last year, is fifth on the list of most active STD. What is the cause of this difference between gonorrhea and syphilis?

I suggest the following explanation: having a round, compact shape, gonorrhea microbes are yang, while syphilis microbes, having a thread-like spiralic shape, are yin. Therefore, gonorrhea microbes are much harder to kill than syphilis microbes. This is the reason that gonorrhea cases outnumbered the cases of syphilis. But since the syphilis microbe is yin, when it does survive the attack of our immune system and/or of antibiotics, it moves into the central, yang organs of the body, that is, the heart and liver, or even deeper into the brain, the central nervous system, and the bones. So, because the weaker – more yin – microbe needs to live in the deeper organs of the body, it is associated with more serious diseases than yang microbes are.

We can summarize these observations as follows:

1. The shape of the microbe tells us whether it is yin or yang: round compact microbes are yang; thread-like microbes are yin.

2. Yin microbes, such as syphilis, are relatively easy to kill, so they account for fewer victims. But when yin microbes do survive in our bodies, they go deep and contribute to very serious disease.

3. Yang microbes, such as gonorrhea, are relatively hard to kill and therefore account for larger numbers of victims. Because these microbes are yang, they are attracted to more yin organs, those nearer to the surface of the body, and so they do less serious damage than yin microbes do.

For instance, according to the 1984 figures, venereal warts claimed twice as many victims as genital herpes did. If we apply to this fact the logic of the three points just mentioned, we can expect that the microbes associated with venereal warts (papilloma virus) are more yang than the microorganisms associated with genital herpes, because we expect the more yang microbe to claim more victims.

We can also expect that, being more yin, the herpes microbe will penetrate into the deeper organs or locations of the body. And this is what we find. As their names indicate, genital herpes shows up within the genitals, and venereal warts appear on the surface of the body.

There is another interesting dimension to this. Venereal warts, associated with the more yang microbe, are more common in women. And genital herpes, associated with the more yin microbe, is more common among men. Since genital herpes is the more yin of the two microorganisms, it contributes to more serious diseases, although both may lead to the appearance of cancer.

The half million 1984 victims of genital herpes brought the total number of sufferers to 20 million adults. Due to its persistent character, herpes has been the most fearful of the STD. Sex partners are terrified of getting herpes. So herpes has been influencing the sex life of the U.S., changing the pattern from sex for pleasure to sex for commitment. However, herpes is not the only disease which is changing the sexual lifestyle of America. We have an even more powerful disease which is changing sex life now. That disease is Acquired Immune Deficiency Syndrome, or AIDS. Since my last article on AIDS in 1983, victims have increased by more than four times. In July of 1983 there were an accounted 1,641 AIDS victims in the U.S. By November of 1984, the number had increased to 6,993. If this rate of increase continues, there will be about two million AIDS victims by 1990.

By that time, AIDS victims will be all over the USA, not only in the big gay communities of New York City or San Francisco. However, this tendency is already on our doorsteps. For example, in a small college town in Northern California with a population of about 50,000, three AIDS victims have died in three years. This number seems to be increasing.

Since AIDS is the most fatal of the sexually transmitted diseases, it is feared as much as cancer is. This fear may change sexual patterns and may bring the long-needed trust between man and woman. If this is the result of AIDS, then it must be a benefactor of mankind, in which case, in my opinion, anyone who tries to manufacture drugs to diminish its symptoms should be punished as an enemy of humanity.

AIDS is presently the most notorious of the sexually transmitted diseases, but all of the STD are gaining ground at an alarming rate. The table shown on page 317 gives only the figures for one year; the total number of people suffering from STD is much higher.

Why this epidemic? What is the cause of these sexually transmitted diseases?

The traditional wisdom of scientists is that gonorrhea is caused by the gonococcus bacteria; syphilis by treponema pallidum (spiral germ); genital herpes by the Herpes Simplex Virus-2 (HSV-2); and AIDS by HTLV-III (the third member of the human T-cell leukemia virus). But from the macrobiotic point of view, neither the viruses nor the bacteria are the causes of sexually transmitted diseases. They never have been. They are the result.

The discovery that bacteria and viruses can only flourish in a body that is already diseased is one of the basic insights of macrobiotics.

The Physical Factor

The bacteria and viruses associated with STD grow best in a warm environment; this is a sign that these microbes are yin. They survive in yin conditions, in liquids – such as fruit sugars – and surrounded by warmth. If they are surrounded by cold, they never grow. If they don't have yin foods, they die.

In other words, a warm environment, yin foods, and, finally, the lack of a healthy immune system are the real causes of STD. And where do these three causes meet? They meet under conditions of sexual promiscuity, of drug use/abuse, where there is poor diet, and in favorable climates. I will explain each of these.

Promiscuity. The promiscuous lifestyle involves excessive sexual intercourse. Semen is made from blood. Therefore, for men, too much sexual intercourse means too much loss of blood, including white cells (the immune system). It has been reported that the average AIDS victim has had sixty different sexual partners in a 12-month period (*Time* magazine, July 4, 1983).

Drug use/abuse. For people of promiscuous lifestyle, sex is just for pleasure and more sex is more pleasure. In order to achieve more and more pleasure through sex, they take sex stimulants, alkyl nitrates. The use of such drugs has a twofold effect on susceptibility to STD.

First, since sex stimulants raise the sex drive they worsen the condition mentioned above – they cause the loss of even more semen and thus deplete the blood of white cells.

The other result of the use of these stimulants is the same condition that any drug use brings, a weakening of the blood. Drugs are acid and very yin, and so they acidify the blood and damage the immune system.

Diet. A diet high in sugar, fruit, yogurt, ice cream, vinegar and/or alcohol, and low in salt makes the blood very yin. Yin blood is a good environment for the growth of microbes, especially those associated with STD. Macrobiotic books or experienced leaders can offer dietary guidance.

Environment. The mechanism of sexually transmitted disease is as follows. Because their nature is yin, the microbes associated with STD live in very warm climates. (A yang climate helps to grow yin creatures, and vice versa.)

People living in a tropical climate, for instance, are surrounded by these microbes and are exposed to them sooner or later even without sex. If these people eat a yang diet – one that is low in sugar and fruit – then their blood is yang and they have a strong immune system, and so they never develop the symptoms of STD, even though they may be carrying STD-associated microbes in their bodies.

When these people of the tropics migrate to a cooler place – a place where tropical microbes have never lived before – many of the microbes they are carrying die due to the change of climate. If, however, the immigrants have sexual intercourse with people of the cooler climate, and if the northerners have weak immune systems, then the tropical bacteria and viruses have access to a perfect place to live, namely the warm, moist organs of the human body such as the sex organs and the anus. This is transmission.

This is also the mechanism by which people from Haiti have brought AIDS into this country.

In other words, as opposed to common belief, a promiscuous lifestyle is not the only cause of any of the STD, even AIDS. The fundamental cause lies deeper, in the conditions of microbial life.

The AIDS microbe is so yin that it prefers to stay in the male sex organs rather than in the female. In this respect AIDS is very much like syphilis, which is also very yin and therefore prefers to live in men's bodies rather than in women's. It is this character of the AIDS virus which is the reason the disease is more common among homosexual people.

However, a yang woman can attract the AIDS virus if she has sexual contact with a man who is carrying the microbe.

In fact, AIDS can probably be transmitted through the air and soil, without any sexual intercourse at all.

George Ohsawa pointed out that although Western medicine thinks that tropical ulcers are sexually transmitted, he found that such ulcers could also be caused by eating a diet rich in fruit and sugar. So you don't need to have sex to have STD.

The Spiritual Factor

We are doing something wrong in modern civilization. We have cancer, AIDS, more and more unknown diseases one after another. Ten years ago we were afraid of the atomic bomb. Then we were afraid of heart attacks. Now we are afraid of cancer. Whether war or disease, we always have something cursing us. There is something wrong in our thinking to cause such troubles.

Do you know what this is called? We call it 'freedom'. We are free to do anything – that's the philosophy of modern civilization. We can do anything we want. That has caused the present civilization, crime, diseases, medicine, and STD.

If we want to go to the moon, we go to the moon. We can put a chimpanzee's heart into a man so as to prolong that man's life for a week. We can have sex with anybody we want.

Since we can do anything, we can eat anything we want. Food companies will manufacture any food which sells and makes a profit. We do have the freedom to do anything, but we also have limitations, especially in foods.

There are misunderstandings of what freedom is. For instance, there is a rumor that in the Himalayas there are saints who live for years without eating. However, even if this rumor is true, the saints could not live for more than several minutes without oxygen.

Freedom exists in our spirit, so that we can think anything. But biologically and physiologically we are unfree. We can wish to eat anything we want. This is spiritual freedom. But we cannot do it. In a dream we can eat a gallon of ice cream, but if we do this in our physical body, then we will be sick.

Once, I ate cheesecake three days in a row. On the fourth day – at my lecture – I lost my voice. I had to confess my greediness to my audience.

This is the same in sex. If we have sex excessively, we will be sick, or at least weakened. People don't realize that there is this limitation. We have a sugar limit, too, and a fat, protein, and salt limit. The limitation is on both sides – too much and too little.

If you are a monkey, you have certain limitations. If you are a horse, you have different limitations. The limitation is different for each species. If you are a fish, you can drink as much as you want all day long. But for a human being it's different.

Macrobiotics amounts to finding the limitations and trying to live within them. And when we are living within our physical limitations, then our spirituality is free. Macrobiotics seeks freedom in spirit. For that we have to first understand the physical limitations. If we act in an unlimited way physically, then our spirituality is limited.

For example, if we indulge excessively in fatty foods, we will be in trouble with heart disease, which then causes very limited living conditions. Discipline is the foundation of spiritual freedom. God didn't give us unlimited freedom biologically and physiologically. But appreciating and taking into consideration our unfree physical condition leads us to greater freedom, both physically and spiritually.

For instance, we can live on this planet until we are maybe eighty years old. Our body temperature should be about

98.6 degrees F. Our body fluid should normally have a pH of 7.4. Our acid/alkaline range has very narrow limitations; that is to say, a pH of 6.9 on the acid end and 7.8 on the alkaline end. At a pH of 6.9 we go into a coma, and at 7.8 we experience epileptic seizure.

Also our blood count is limited. And we have to have a certain blood pressure. Too high or low is no good. As human beings, we have limitations everywhere. But our spiritual activities are not limited.

When our spirit is in Infinity, our happiness is infinite. But most people stay in the limited, unfree world, because they are living with emotion or ego and not spirit. Emotions are also limited – even joy and happiness. If we have too much joy, it can change into sadness. When you have joy, you have to know its limitations. If you are angry at your limitations, then you are bound in the limited world and will be unhappy. If you appreciate your limitations, then you are in the world of spirit, of freedom.

For example, sickness. Sickness is a sign that you are limited. Not realizing this, most people continue to act freely. Then sickness becomes more severe until they realize their limitations. Some people who reach this point then change their diet or lifestyle. The point of macrobiotic education is to realize for ourselves that we are physically limited.

This is the cultivation of humbleness. When we think that we can do anything we want, we become arrogant. This arrogance causes sickness.

So-called freedom is another name for arrogance. Western civilization has been after freedom for many years. However, its freedom was arrogance and so it has made people unfree with many diseases. As long as we have the arrogance of freedom we will continue to have diseases.

Modern medicine arrogantly tries to conquer those diseases, but we always have more new ones and the newer diseases are harder to cure than the older ones. Because we are arrogant!

In my opinion, STD comes from the misunderstanding of freedom, from arrogance. When we have pain, we are free to kill the virus or bacteria. We can change sex partners as many times as we want. We can have sex as many times as we want. This idea of freedom is the cause of STD.

Supreme Judgment

To live is to act. Action is determined by our thinking or judgment. Sound and right thinking leads us to good action, which in turn leads us to health and happiness. Therefore, it is imperative to improve our thinking or judgment as much as possible. According to Ohsawa, in order to achieve eternal happiness we have to attain supreme judgment. For many years I have tried to answer the question of how to attain supreme judgment. Here is my preliminary report on this difficult question.

When we were born we had almost no activity of consciousness except those subconscious actions by which the baby sucks the mother's milk and cries when hungry. This is the stage of mechanical, blind judgment or intuitive consciousness. This judgment can be performed without the big brain; it follows the lower part of the brain – the corpus callosum, thalamus, hypothalamus, the brain stem, and the central and peripheral nervous systems.

About forty days after birth the baby begins to see and then to hear. This is the beginning of sensorial judgment. A little later the baby can notice smells and recognize the taste of foods and other things. At this time the baby can distinguish shapes, colors, sounds, etc. This level of judgment is mainly a function of the parietal lobe of the brain.

About two months after birth the baby starts to show

volitions and emotions. (Compared to other babies, macrobiotic babies are calmer and less hyperactive, so they are easier to take care of.) This is the beginning of emotional judgment, due to the development of the occipital lobe of the brain.

When the mechanical, sensorial, and emotional stages of judgment are completely developed, the fourth or intellectual judgment begins: recognizing, comparing, and distinguishing differences between things. The temporal lobe of the brain is active in this kind of judgment. Intellectual judgment normally begins around the age of four. At this stage children even start having the concept of numbers. At first, they recognize one. If you give them several things, they hold only one at a time. Next they recognize two and then many. Later they recognize numbers larger than two – probably around six years old.

The intellectual judgment develops very fast around this age. Children ask many questions which their mothers often think are meaningless, unimaginable, or unanswerable: Why is the sky blue? Why are leaves green? Why isn't this road or hill flat? Why are mountains high? Why is ocean water salty? Who makes the ocean waves? and so on. Busy mothers usually ask the children to be quiet, and thus stop their children's intellectual development.

The young Charles Kettering asked his mother one day, "Why are plant leaves green?" His mother replied, "I don't know, son; please find out for yourself." Instead of discouraging the boy's intellectual activity, Charles's mother encouraged it. And because of his mother's encouragement this boy continued to search for the reason that plants are green. Much later he established the C.F. Kettering Foundation, where scientists identified chlorophyll as the cause of the green in plants.

A very important judgment starts to develop around the age of six: social and economic judgment. Children are very social at this age and they want to conform with others. On the first day my daughter went to elementary school, my wife gave her a peanut butter sandwich on whole wheat bread for her lunch. She came back home without eating at school because the other students had told her that her sandwich was bad and strange. She was conforming to the other children. When I was of school age, I was living in a poor neighborhood of downtown Tokyo. My adoptive father, a successful businessman, was rich, so mother bought me an overcoat for the cold winter. But since none of my classmates had such a coat to wear, I didn't want to wear it. I was ashamed to be different. This is the beginning of social judgment.

The economic part of this level of judgment may start a little later than the social, depending on one's living conditions. If one grows up in a poor family, economic judgment may develop sooner. Social and economic judgment taken together are the fifth stage of judgment.

After one has fully developed the first five stages of judgment, one's judgment raises one level higher to the sixth: ideological or religious judgment. This is the judgment of good and bad. Some religions, including Christianity, seem to be based on the concept that man is bad and needs the love or mercy of a savior. There are completely opposite ones, such as the Zen sect of Buddhism or the Japanese Shinto religion, which say that man is good, or even that man is a god.

From the first to the sixth, each of these stages of consciousness represent dualism or relative thinking. Therefore, there is no absolute and eternal truth, happiness, or judgment in these stages. Antagonism always arises. This is not absolute. It is relative. People are seeking eternal happiness and absolute righteousness in the world of relative judgment. Thus they cannot find it. There is always brutal fighting, even among religious groups, scientific theories are constantly replaced by new ones, and many marriages are broken so soon and so often.

One must reach supreme judgment, the seventh level, which is absolute and universal love that embraces everything and turns every antagonism into complementarity.

Supreme judgment is the same as Infinity, Oneness, or God. This is the reason we can embrace everything and turn antagonism into complementarity whenever we reach supreme judgment. Only then do we have eternal happiness, because in the lower six stages of judgment our thinking creates antagonism, shortcomings, and disputes. People commonly say that they are raising judgment when they progress from a lower to a higher level, such as from the second to the fourth level. However, this raising of judgment is only relative and of little importance. Reaching supreme judgment is the real raising of judgment.

In order to raise judgment or consciousness, you must have a map of judgment. The spiral drawing is a map of the infinite universe and also a map of absolute judgment (or universal consciousness), which also includes dualistic and relative thinking.

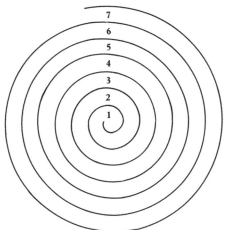

7th Stage: supreme judgment
6th Stage: religious judgment
5th Stage: social judgment
4th Stage: intellectual judgment
3rd Stage: emotional judgment
2nd Stage: sensorial judgment
1st Stage: mechanical judgment

As you can see in the drawing, the lower judgments are

located inside of the higher judgments. In other words, the lower judgments are more yang than the higher, or the higher judgments are more yin than the lower. Therefore, raising judgment means to yinnize judgment or consciousness (without yinnizing the body too much).

How can we yinnize our judgment?

First, by giving up what we like: detachment from our sensorial or emotional judgments. As soon as we detach from our lower judgments such as wanting to eat ice cream, wanting to buy a nice car, wanting to marry a beautiful woman (at any cost), etc., we will be at the supreme judgment.

You may have begun following the macrobiotic principles by giving up some of the sensorial judgments, such as eating meat, candy, lots of fruit, etc. This giving up of sensorial likings was a manifestation of supreme judgment. When supreme judgment reveals itself, your mind is at peace and all metabolic and hormonal processes are smooth and in order. This peace of mind together with the macrobiotic diet is what improved your health. Your health did not improve by the diet alone.

A while later you stop giving up what you liked. Rather, you give up the delicious macrobiotic meals and you fall again to the lower judgment of the sensorial level. This sensorial judgment will create questions, doubts, and complaints; that is to say, many emotional hangups. This destroys peace of mind and disrupts the smooth functioning of metabolism and hormone secretion. Then health improvement stops. This explains why many macrobiotic students improve their health so much at first and later stop improving. [This is also explained in *How Change Changes*.]

The other way to reach supreme judgment is to give: give what you want most, in order to help others. Helping others is a manifestation of love, and love is the state of supreme judgment. This love or supreme judgment makes it easy for one to give up sensorial or sentimental things. For example, the Japanese often give up eating favorite foods, such as fish, in order to cure the sickness of a loved one. It is hard to give up foods you like, but it is easier if you do this for others because you are doing so with love, with higher judgment if not supreme judgment.

In my opinion, these two – detachment and giving – are the most effective ways to raise our judgment.

However, no matter how much we succeed in reaching supreme judgment, we will not stay there for long. We may stay with it for only a second. We may even stay a day or so. But even if we have supreme judgment just a short time, it has tremendous power for our well-being and happiness, for at that moment we are Infinity and the world of God and Love. By repeating this up-and-down experience, we will climb up the ladder of judgment and be able to stay at supreme judgment longer.

Index

Grayslake Area Public Library District
Grayslake, Illinois

1. A fine will be charged on each book which is not returned when it is due.

2. All injuries to books beyond reasonable wear and all losses shall be made good to the satisfaction of the Librarian.

3. Each borrower is held responsible for all books drawn on his card and for all fines accruing on the same.

Dear Parent:
Your child's love of reading starts here!

Every child learns to read in a different way and at his or her own speed. Some go back and forth between reading levels and read favorite books again and again. Others read through each level in order. You can help your young reader improve and become more confident by encouraging his or her own interests and abilities. From books your child reads with you to the first books he or she reads alone, there are I Can Read Books for every stage of reading:

SHARED READING
Basic language, word repetition, and whimsical illustrations, ideal for sharing with your emergent reader

BEGINNING READING
Short sentences, familiar words, and simple concepts for children eager to read on their own

READING WITH HELP
Engaging stories, longer sentences, and language play for developing readers

READING ALONE
Complex plots, challenging vocabulary, and high-interest topics for the independent reader

ADVANCED READING
Short paragraphs, chapters, and exciting themes for the perfect bridge to chapter books

I Can Read Books have introduced children to the joy of reading since 1957. Featuring award-winning authors and illustrators and a fabulous cast of beloved characters, I Can Read Books set the standard for beginning readers.

A lifetime of discovery begins with the magical words **"I Can Read!"**

Visit www.icanread.com for information
on enriching your child's reading experience.

I Can Read Book® is a trademark of HarperCollins Publishers.

Sid the Science Kid: What's that Smell?
™ & © 2010 The Jim Henson Company. JIM HENSON'S mark & logo, SID THE SCIENCE KID mark & logo,
characters and elements are trademarks of The Jim Henson Company.
All Rights Reserved. Manufactured in China.
No part of this book may be used or reproduced in any manner whatsoever without written permission
except in the case of brief quotations embodied in critical articles and reviews. For information address
HarperCollins Children's Books, a division of HarperCollins Publishers, 10 East 53rd Street, New York, NY 10022.
www.icanread.com

Library of Congress catalog card number: 2009939635
ISBN 978-0-06-185259-6

Typography by Rick Farley
11 12 13 SCP 10 9 8 7 6 5 4 3
❖
First Edition

I Can Read!

BEGINNING READING 1

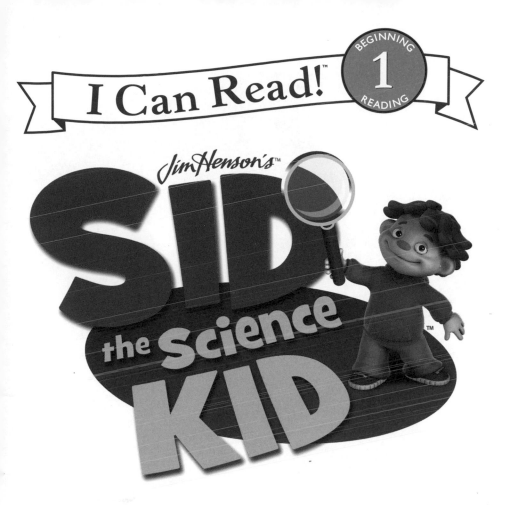

Jim Henson's™

SID the Science KID™

What's that Smell?

by Jennifer Frantz

HARPER

An Imprint of HarperCollins*Publishers*

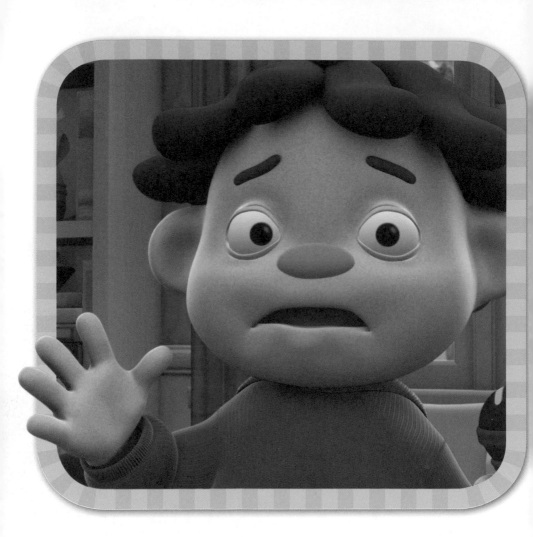

"Ew! I smell something
not so good," said Sid.
"It's my baby brother
Zeke's diaper!"

4

"Breakfast is almost ready,"

said Mom.

She carried Zeke to the kitchen.

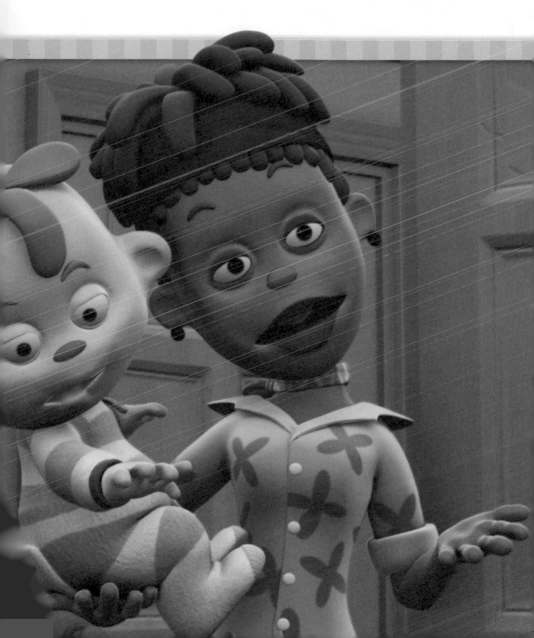

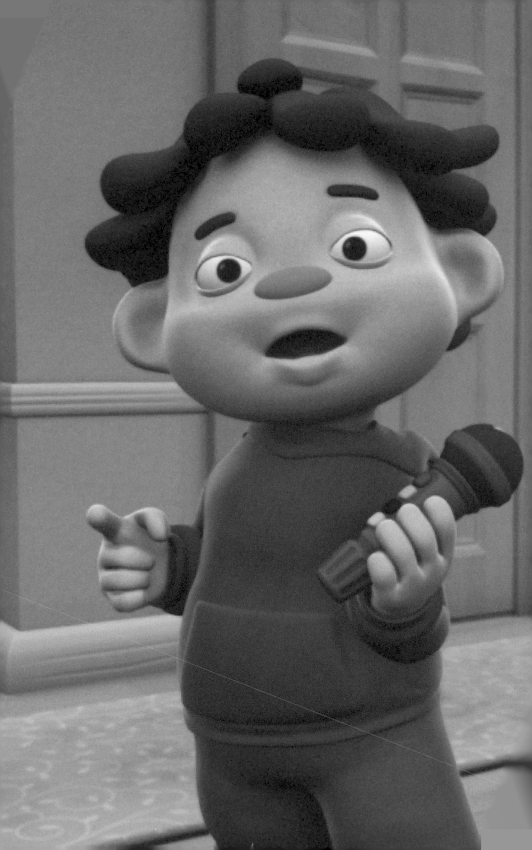

"Icky!" said Sid.

"If Zeke is in the kitchen now,

how can I still smell him?

What's the big idea?

How can you smell things

that are far away?"

Sid wanted to know.

"Mom," said Sid.
"Do you notice
a funny smell
coming from Zeke?"

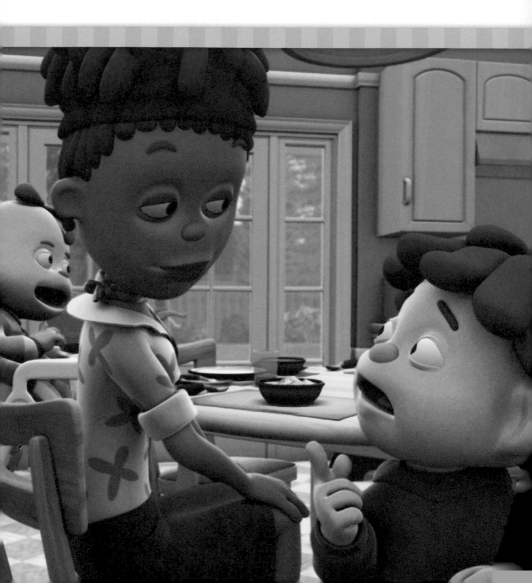

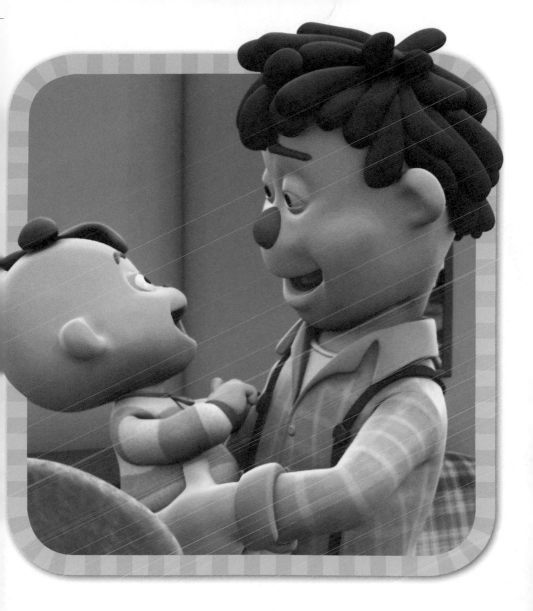

"Ooh! Dirty diaper,"

said Dad.

"I'm on it."

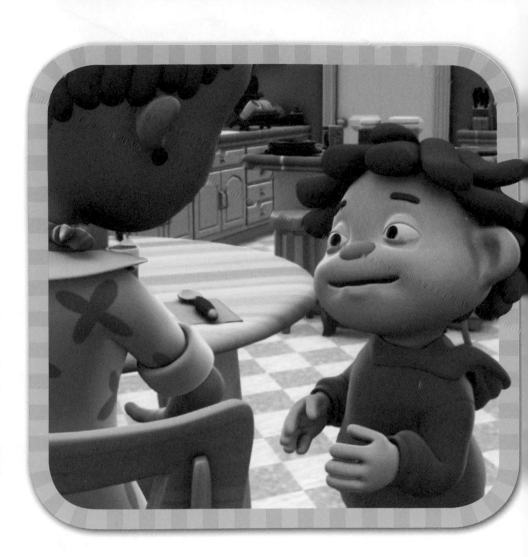

"How could I smell
Zeke's diaper from
down the hall?"
said Sid.

10

"You know," said Mom.
"Zeke's diaper isn't
the only thing you can smell
from far away."

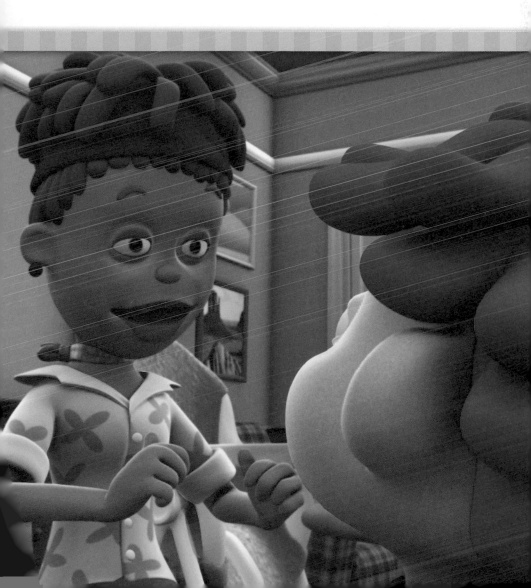

Sid closed his eyes.
"You're right," he said.
"I can smell Dad's
famous pancakes!"

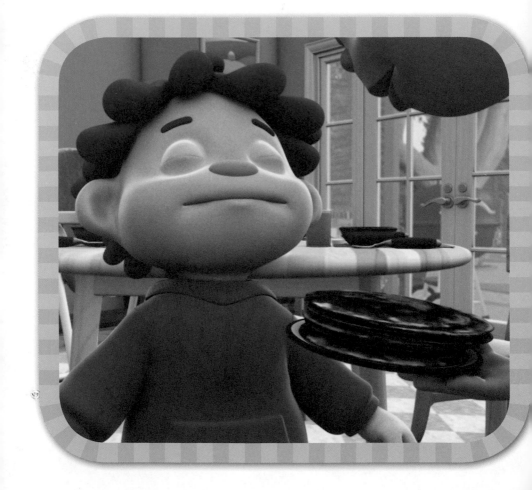

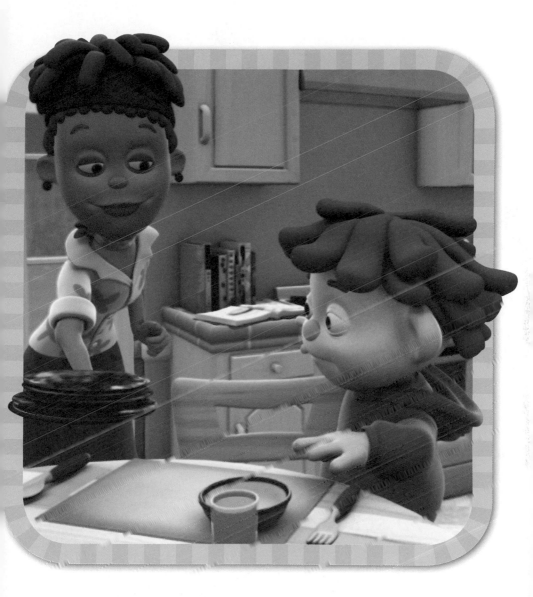

"Good!" said Mom.

"It's time to eat breakfast
before you're late for school."

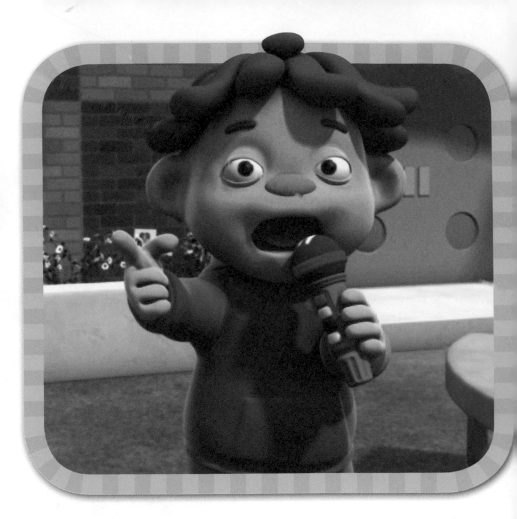

At school, Sid asked
his friends about smells.
"Have you ever smelled
something that was far away?"
he said.

"Yes," said May.

"We have flowers in our garden that I can smell inside our house."

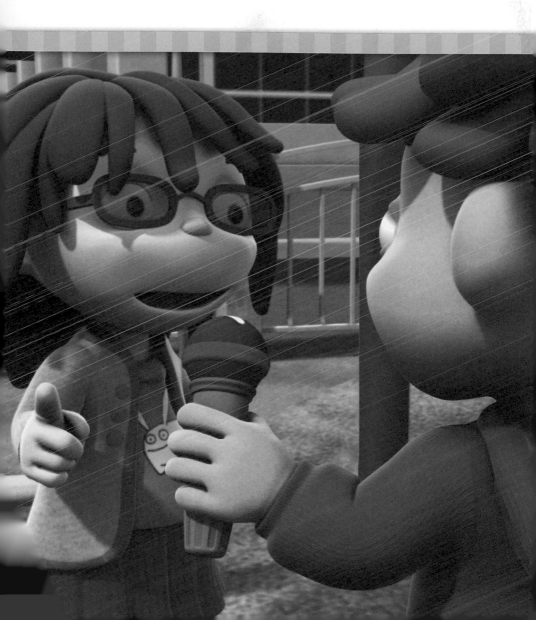

"My aunt Peggy made
a blueberry pie," said Gerald.
"I could smell it from
across the kitchen."

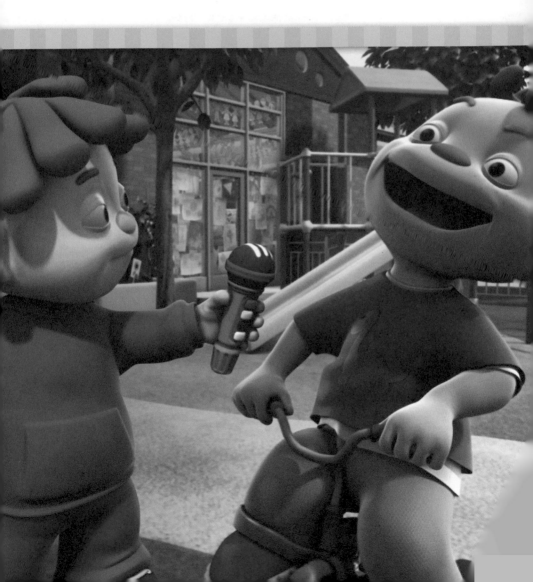

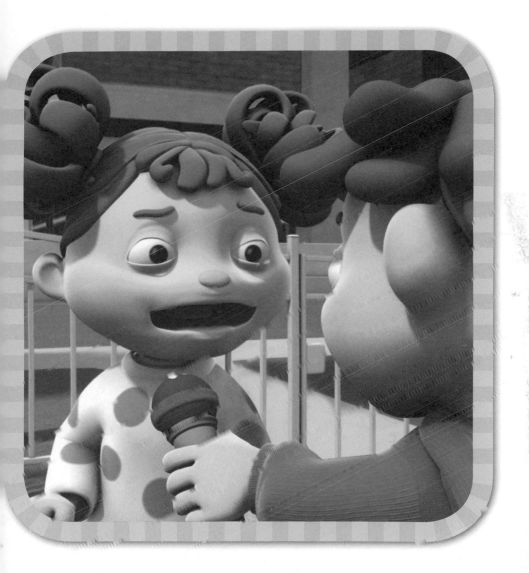

"My uncle Roy's feet,"

said Gabricla.

"He has smelly socks. Yuck!"

"Come on in!"
said Teacher Susie.
"It's rug time."

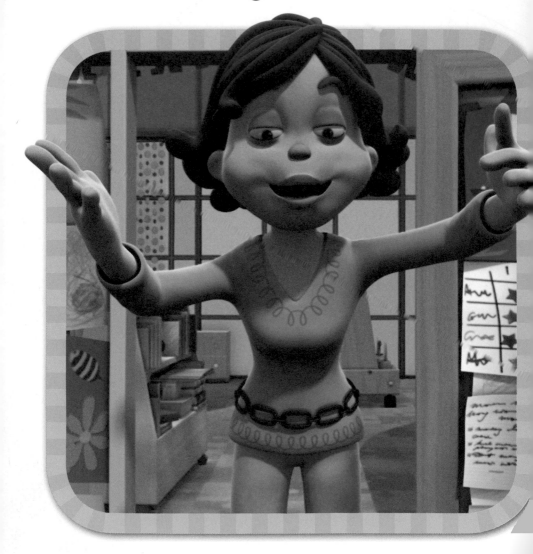

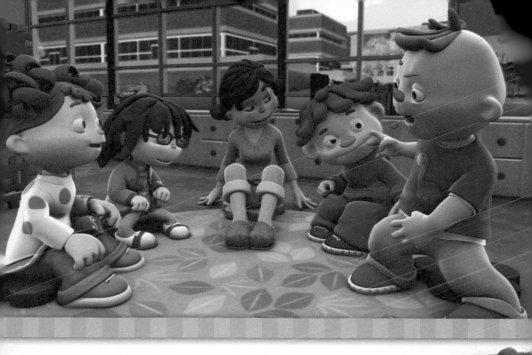

Everyone sat on the rug.

"We were talking

about smelling things

that are far away," said May.

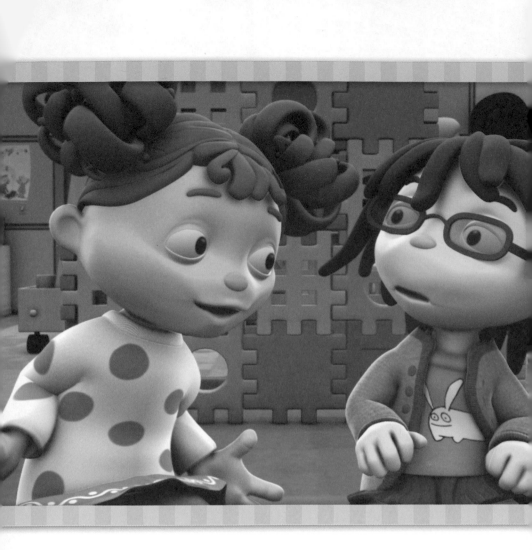

"Does the wind blow smells around?"
said Gabriela.

"Close!" said Teacher Susie.

"Smells are teeny tiny things
called molecules," said Teacher Susie.
"They can travel in the air,
even without wind.
Then they land in your nose."

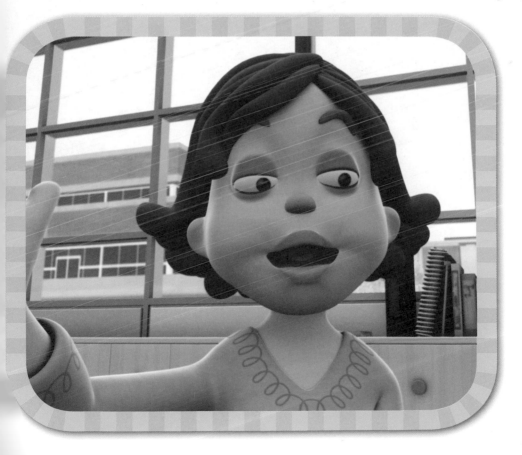

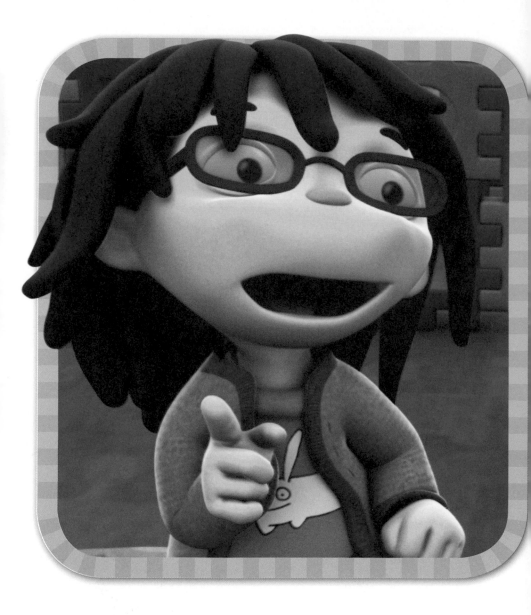

"I don't see any molecules,"

said May.

"Molecules are too small to see with our eyes," said Teacher Susie. "We use our noses to smell them. That's our sense of smell!"

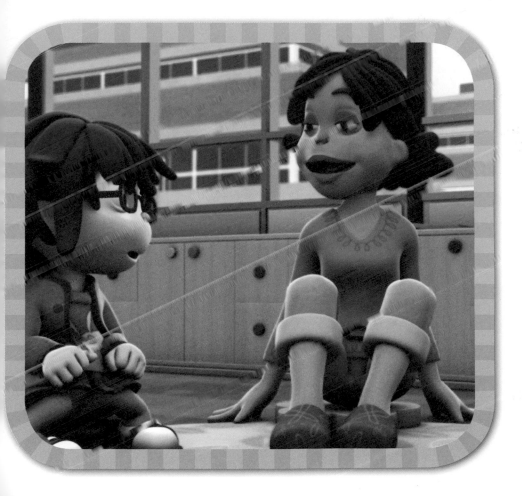

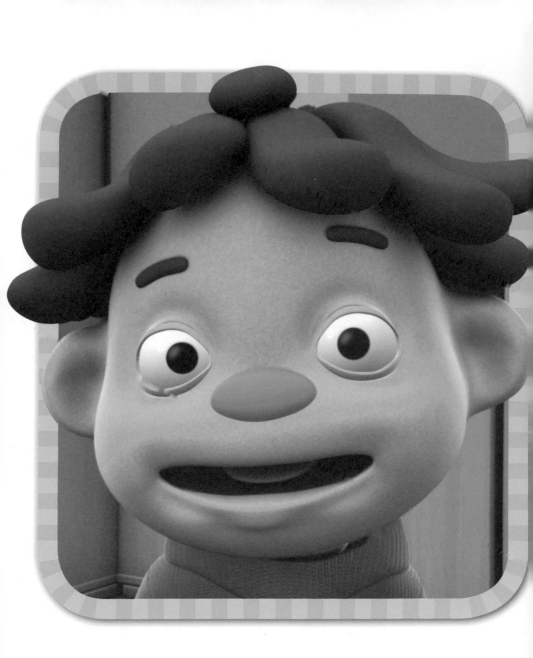

"Wow," said Sid.

"So that's how we smell!"

"That's right!" said Teacher Susie.
"Let's take our noses
to the Super Fab Lab
to find out more."

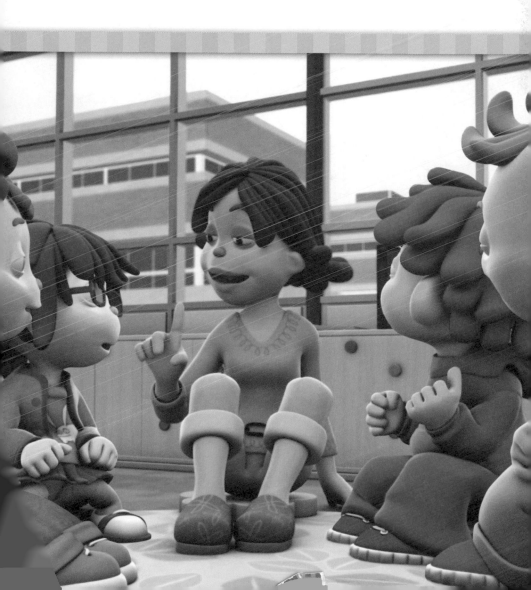

"No peeking!" said Teacher Susie.

"Each cup has food in it.

Guess what food you smell."

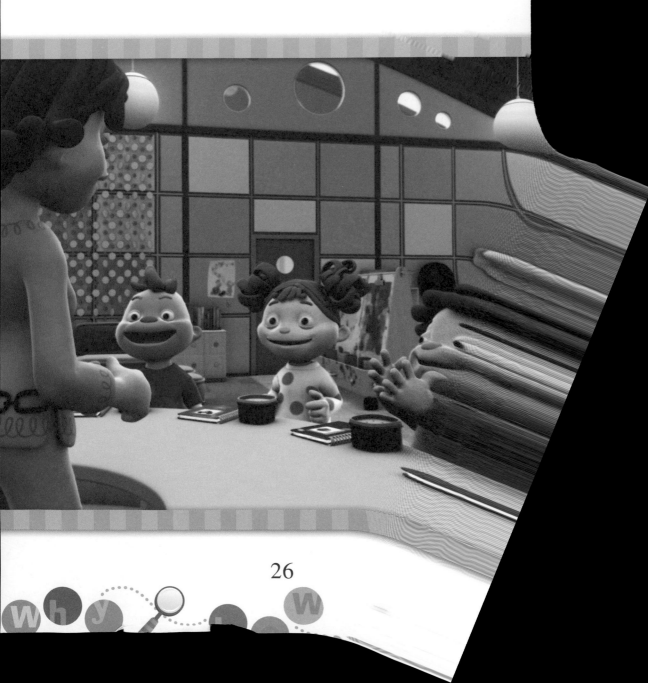

"That's right!" said Teacher Susie.
"Let's take our noses
to the Super Fab Lab
to find out more."

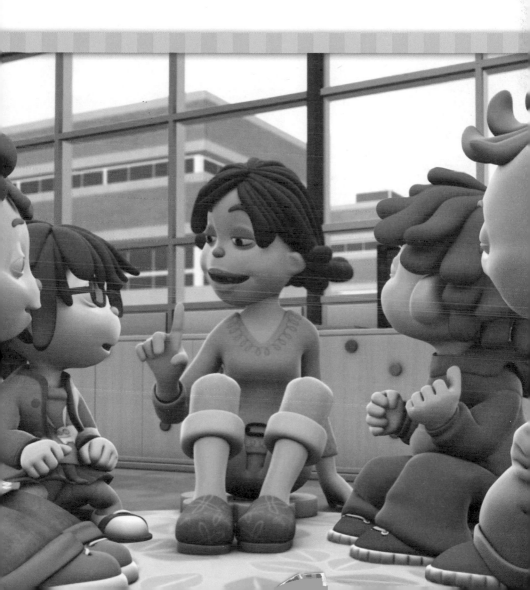

"No peeking!" said Teacher Susie.

"Each cup has food in it.

Guess what food you smell."

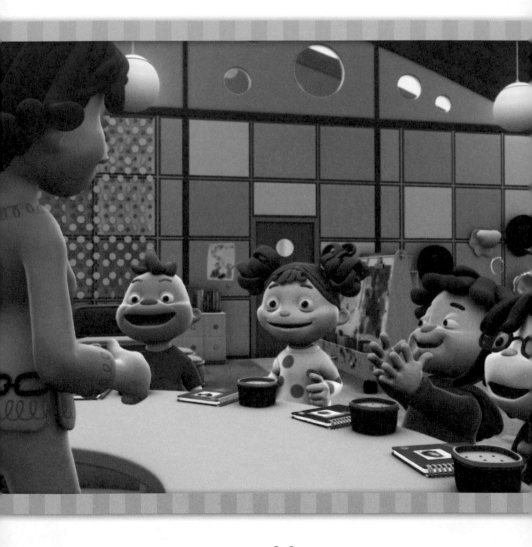

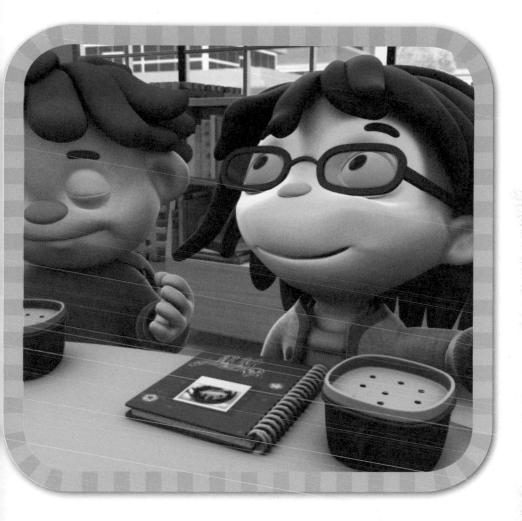

"Mmm, this one smells
like grandma's cookies,"
said May.
"Cinnamon!"

27

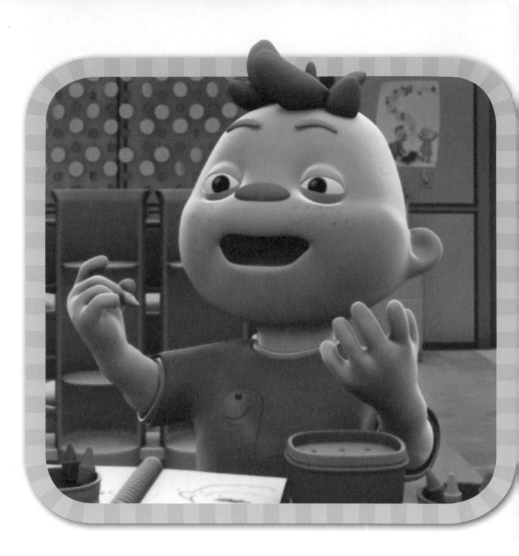

"This one smells
like the movies,"
said Gerald.
"It's popcorn."

28

"This one smells
a little spicy," said Sid.
"Is it mustard?"
"Nope," said Gabriela.
"It's onions."

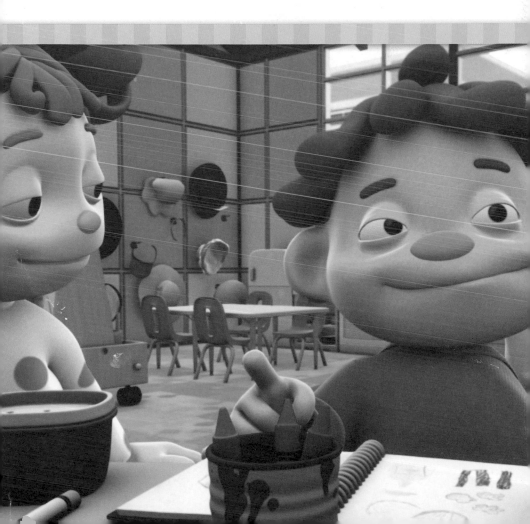

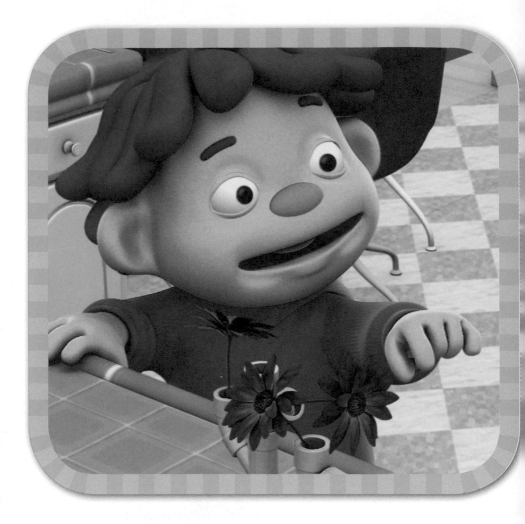

Back at home,

Sid smelled something nice

coming from the kitchen.

"Flowers!" he said.

"Good job, nose," said Sid.
"I'm sure glad you can
smell molecules . . .
even ones from stinky diapers!"

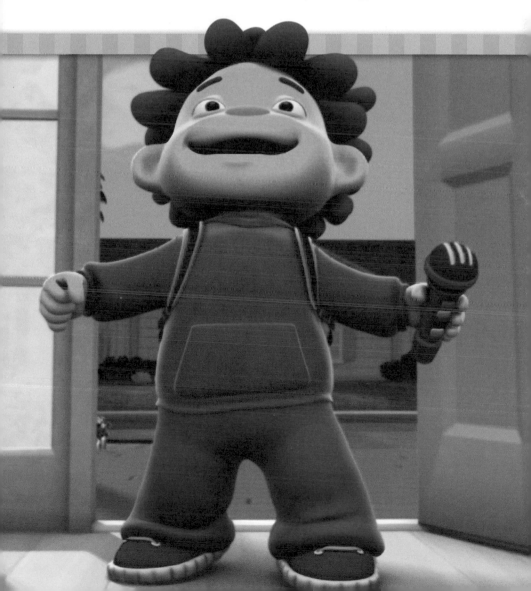

LAUGHTERNOON
a good time for some smelly jokes

What did one eye say to the other eye?

Don't look now, but something between us smells.

What is something you can watch that also smells?

Smell-evision!

How do you stop a fish from smelling?

You hold his nose.